Anal
SEX
BASICS

MW01000206

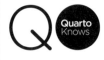

Quarto is the authority on a wide range of topics.

Quarto educates, entertains and enriches the lives of
our readers—enthusiasts and lovers of hands-on living.

www.QuartoKnows.com

© 2016 Quarto Publishing Group USA Inc.
Text © 2016 Quarto Publishing Group USA Inc.
Illustrations © 2016 Quarto Publishing Group
USA Inc.

First published in the USA in 2016 by
Fair Winds Press, an imprint of
Quarto Publishing Group USA Inc.
100 Cummings Center
Suite 406-L
Beverly, MA 01915-6101
www.QuartoKnows.com

All rights reserved. No part of this book may
be reproduced or utilized, in any form or by
any means, electronic or mechanical, without
prior permission in writing from the publisher.

The Publisher maintains the records relating
to images in this book required by 18 USC
2257. Records are located at Rockport
Publishers, Inc., 100 Cummings Center, Suite
406-L, Beverly, MA 01915-6101.

18 17 16 15 14   1 2 3 4 5

ISBN: 978-1-59233-703-3

Digital edition published in 2016
eISBN: 978-1-62788-828-8

Library of Congress Cataloging-in-Publication
Data available

Cover design: Burge Agency
Book design: Burge Agency
Illustrations: Laia Albaladejo
Photography: Shutterstock.com
Developmental editing: Megan Buckley

Printed and bound in Hong Kong

Anal

SEX

BASICS

THE BEGINNER'S GUIDE TO MAXIMIZING ANAL PLEASURE FOR EVERY BODY

Carlyle Jansen

FAIR WINDS

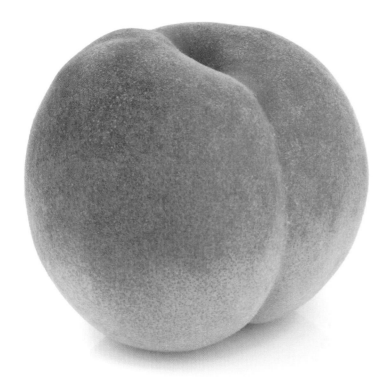

TO THOSE WHO BELIEVE THAT THERE IS ALWAYS MORE POTENTIAL FOR PLEASURE, I HOPE THAT THIS BOOK EDUCATES, ILLUMINATES, AND INSPIRES YOU TO HONOR AND LOVE YOUR BUTT IN WHICHEVER WAYS YOU CHOOSE.

—CARLYLE JANSEN

CONTENTS

CHOOSE YOUR
ANAL ADVENTURE

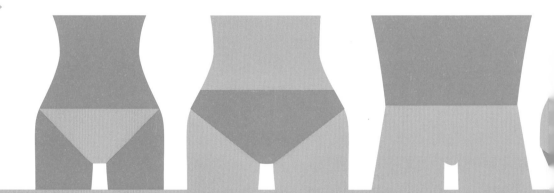

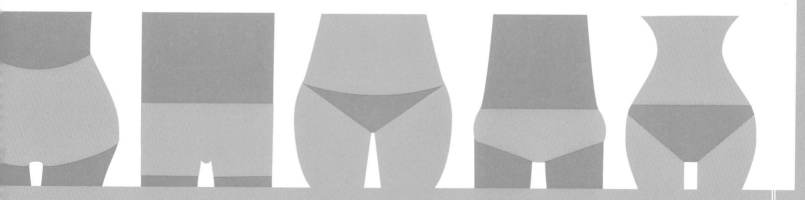

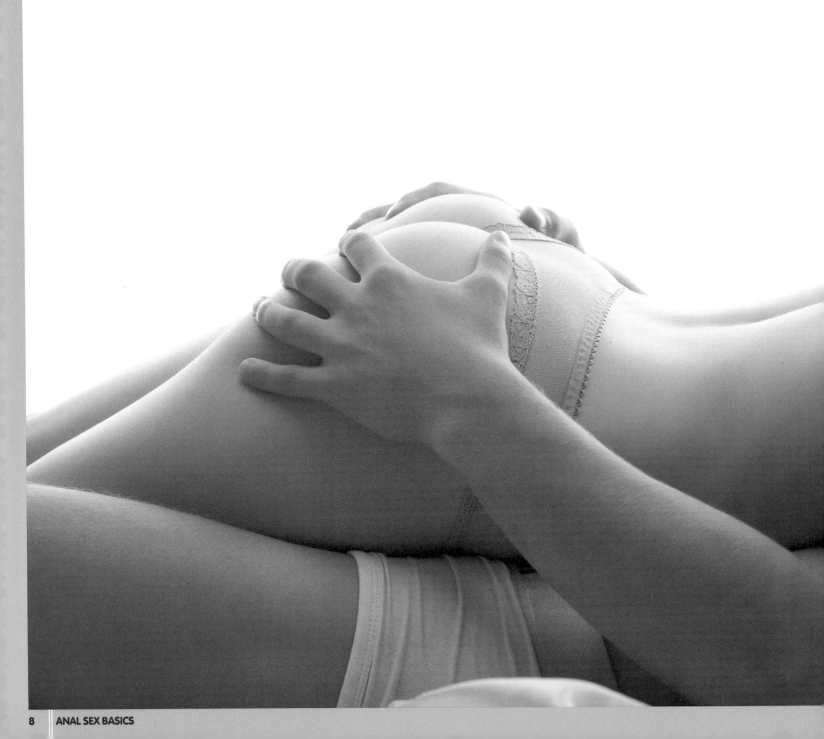

INTRODUCTION

Welcome to your anal adventure. Whether you have experienced amazing anal pleasure already, you have had unpleasant previous encounters but are looking to try again with better success, or you're not so sure whether you actually want to take the anal plunge, this book will help you navigate your options and make the best decisions for how and how far you wish to proceed.

My sexual adventure started many years ago. At the time, I was not very comfortable with sex at all. My family did not discuss it, and when my class had a sex discussion at school in tenth grade, I was horrified to think that others might already be doing it. I wasn't ready to take the plunge into sex until I was twenty-one. Masturbation had not even been on my radar at that point. My first partner quickly learned that I was not able to orgasm. Once, my partner stopped what he was doing and asked me what I liked. "Aren't you supposed to know that?" I replied. Gently, he suggested that it might be helpful if I knew a little more about my own body and about what brought me pleasure.

After two years of little success in finding orgasm on my own or with a partner, I gave up, resigning myself to the idea that some people are tall, others are short; and some can do math, others are better at art; and some can orgasm, others can't. I was fine with my nonorgasmic status until, several years and relationships later, I was dumped. My inability to orgasm was getting in the way of my relationships. A good friend suggested I try a vibrator, the Hitachi Magic Wand. It did the trick, and I was now part of the orgasmic club. Finally, I knew what the fuss was all about, and I decided it was high time I really learned about sex.

Living in Seattle at the time, I started my sexual awakening. I discovered the Body Electric School. Though the school's workshops were originally for men only, I attended the first of its sessions for women. There, I found boundless opportunities for and types of pleasure that I could explore. I was hungry for sexual knowledge and experience. Anal play was not a specific interest of mine, but it was on the menu so I decided to sample it.

Chester Maynard was the guru of anal play, and I was one of the many who had the privilege of attending a few of his workshops. During his lifetime, he passed along many amazing tips and techniques to those open to expanding their erotic repertoires and pleasure potential. He taught thousands of men and many women about enhancing anal pleasure. From him I learned how to give and receive anal pleasure in ways that I had

Our Survey

In order to add a diversity of voices to this book, beginners and seasoned anal players were recruited to share their experiences with anal pleasure. Some were given an instructional DVD on anal massage by Erospirit and tested new toys, as well as reviewing any already in their collection. They were asked to comment on their experiences and preferences with toys, cleaning, preparation, cleanup and aftercare, positions, communication, prostate play, kink, and any advice that they wanted to pass on to you!

FROM OUR SURVEY

" *I use my knowledge of my body, my diet, and my health as a barometer of whether or not I want something in my ass. If anything seems off, then the area is off-limits.* "

never imagined were possible. He certainly expanded the definition of *anal play* beyond "penis in butt."

Anal play is the fastest way to uncover someone's emotional mind-set. This area of the body stores tension (hence the term "anal-retentive" as well as other sentiments). For some, anal play can arouse immense pleasure and other powerful (sometimes negative) feelings. Whether it is emotionally potent or just wildly fun, anal stimulation can lead to intimate, intense, and incredible erotic play.

Anal sex evokes a variety of connotations, assumptions, and reactions—negative and positive. One might assume it merely means "penis-in-butt" sex. But according to Jack Morin, author of *Anal Pleasure and Health* (2010), anal intercourse is the *least* common form of anal pleasure most people engage in. More folks enjoy external play and the insertion of toys or fingers than insertion of a penis.

We've been led to associate anal sex with pain; after all, it's an activity in an area of the body we've been taught to stay away from since childhood. Often people fear infections, HIV, and AIDS as a result of anal play. My goal in this book is to help you move past these assumptions and associations with anal sex. I'll address these fears and misconceptions and offer a broader snapshot of the pleasures and possibilities of anal play. I hope that you will gain a more complete understanding of why folks enjoy it, how to play safely, and tips to make it a fantastic experience for everyone involved.

This book is for everybody and for every body. It's written to include all bodies, sexes, genders, orientations, desires, and preferences. My goal is that you, no matter who you are, will feel that this book speaks to you. After all, the anus is the equal-opportunity orifice. Just about everyone has one. The principles and pleasures of anal play are very similar, no matter who you are. Anyone can find joy in his or her own or a partner's anus.

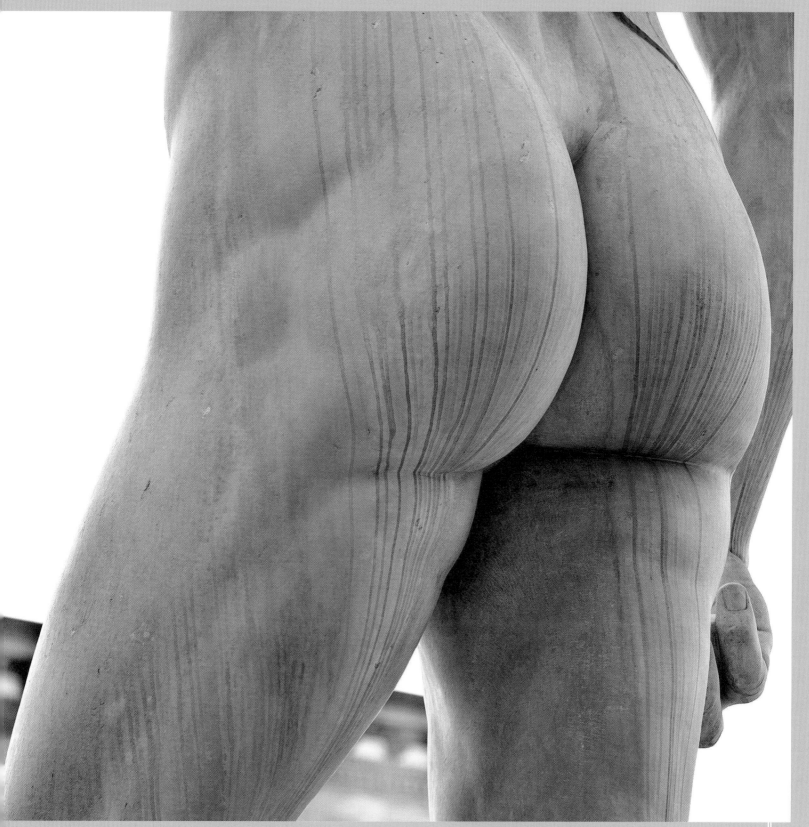

The path to anal sex at this point in my life is the same feeling I had when I was eighteen and lost my virginity: Everybody's doing it—it must be great!

This is your opportunity to try new and exciting forms of pleasure. My hope is that you will be clear with yourself and your partner(s) about your intentions for engaging in anal play. I'm here to help you with that! Communication is always an important skill for all aspects of relationships, but many of us don't feel confident in expressing our desires, fears, and reservations without creating disharmony in the relationship. I'll offer skills to help you communicate what you want, from initiating a conversation to the finer details of pleasure in the midst of anal passion! Chapter 6 will offer you plenty of practical tools to help you craft conversations that lead to enjoying the anal sex you desire.

Perhaps your partner has been begging you to try anal sex. But alternatively, I often hear, "I just want to get a toy/finger in there," as a goal for progressing toward anal sex. If you've had this thought, I encourage you to reframe your goal to focus on pleasure rather than an activity. You may not realize how much pleasure you can get from stimulating all areas of your butt! In subsequent chapters, I hope to impress upon you that you can have great anal sex, even without penetration. Whether you want full-fledged penetration or some exciting play, learn the small steps you can take on your journey, and take them at a speed that suits you both.

You may be put off by the taboo of anal sex. Please remember that many acceptable sex acts today—such as oral sex and masturbation—were taboo only a few decades ago. A taboo is a societal construct, and those change. Anal play may well be the next type of sex that "everyone is doing." For some, the forbidden nature of a taboo gives it that extra-exciting flavor. The rush we gain from doing something a little naughty might be what makes it all the more appealing!

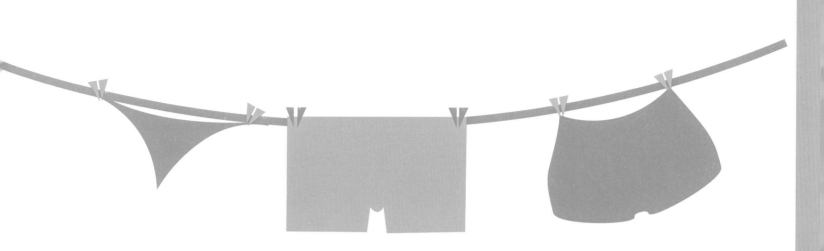

Our language falls into step with the idea of taboos. After all, calling someone an "asshole" is not generally a compliment. Language like this makes it is harder to embrace playing with a part of the body being cast in a negative and dirty light in more than one way. Moreover, most of us do not know what our beloved rosebuds (anuses) look like. It is hard to let someone else play with and view a part of our body that we can't easily see ourselves. Is it clean? Cute? Hairy? Evenly colored? All of these concerns are easily alleviated with the ancient technology of a mirror. Have a look so that you can admire your own beauty and feel better about someone else doing the same!

Finally, anal sex forces us to come to terms with something we would rather not ever have to deal with: poop. But let's face it—farting and pooping are part of life. Don't forget that shit is what fertilizes the earth. If we can shift our thinking to poop as resourceful and life giving, we can develop a whole new relationship with it and with our bodies.

Let's extol the many virtues of and reasons folks engage in anal sex. For one, it can be an extremely powerful form of pleasure. It can offer explosive orgasms to people of all sexes, but especially those with prostates. Many find that playing with their anuses takes them to a new frontier of intimacy that offers deep emotional satisfaction and connection as well as physical pleasure. It is also a way for those with only one hole in their pelvic regions to receive penetration. Anal strap-on sex is a great way to switch roles for some couples or add variety for others. And of course it is always fun to add a little diversity to our sex play and have even more options available to pursue.

If you are interested in embarking in anal pleasure, you are not alone. Studies have shown a proportional increase in anal sex participation over the years. In a 2010 survey led by Debby Herbenick of almost six thousand mostly heterosexual men and women in the United States, approximately 20 percent of women ages eighteen to thirty-nine and 25 percent of men ages twenty-five to forty-nine reported engaging in anal sex in the past year (details available here: www.nationalsexstudy.indiana.edu). Up to 45 percent of men and women have tried it at least once. These numbers have increased since the 1990s, when only 25 percent to 33 percent of young women and men had tried anal sex at least once. You can imagine that the frequency of anal sex is likely underreported; these numbers may be higher in reality.

Whatever your motivation, I hope that this book will help erase any stigma around anal play and that these pages will help you find the depth and pleasure you are looking for. Take it slowly and enjoy the journey. It's better to appreciate the experience gradually and relish the excitement that leaves you wanting more than to have a negative experience that crosses anal sex off the list forever. Many believe that—especially when it comes to anal play—the slower you go, the faster and happier you get there. There is always a next time. Keep the anticipation and the options flowing for the hottest sex you've ever had!

Chapter 1

MYTHS AND PLEASURES:
THE TRUTH ABOUT ANAL SEX

For many of us, our bodies are sources of mystery—and sometimes even fear. When we're young, we're rarely taught about our erogenous zones and how to explore them, and even our knowledge of the basics of reproduction might be limited. So most of our sexual exploration begins by accident in the bathtub, while using the washroom, or when we become sexually active for the first time. And when we do learn about sex, we learn that it works one way and one way only: Penises enter vaginas. End of story. But this oversimplified model is so restrictive that it omits many partner configurations, erogenous zones, and possibilities of play. It also helps to perpetuate the (many!) myths about sex that have emerged from—or have even been created by—interpretations of religious teachings and sex-negative norms and fears, especially when it comes to sexual activities outside of procreation-based vaginal intercourse. Masturbation, for example, has gotten an especially bad rap since time immemorial—and particularly in the nineteenth century, when the so-called medical professionals of the day preached that it could trigger diseases like epilepsy and could cause blindness, hysteria, or reduced sexual desire. Meanwhile, cultural norms also discouraged masturbation. Being "too sexual" could slash your status on the marriage market, especially if you were a woman.

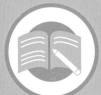

What's in a name?

The word *masturbation* is believed to originate from the Latin words *manus*, or "hand," and *stuprare*, "to defile yourself." So masturbation can be loosely translated as "to defile yourself with your hand"—a pejorative phrase that hardly puts you in the mood for self-love! It's just another example of how language influences the interpretation of the actions it describes.

Like masturbation, anal sex isn't necessary for reproduction. It's been much maligned over the years, and that means the facts about anal sex—including cleanliness, safety, and exactly who engages in it—have been twisted. Thus, it's been driven underground. In fact, it's still technically an illegal activity in many American states and in a number of countries around the world. That just isn't fair. Of course, when it comes to sex, it's important to stay safe, just as it's important to be mindful of safety in other aspects of life. For example, we tell our kids to cross the street at the crosswalk, to stay away from chemicals, and not to touch other people's "private parts." But with experience and maturity, we learn that there are relatively safe ways to cross the street without a convenient intersection; we're able to use chemicals for photography or science experiments without hurting ourselves; and we respectfully and consensually explore private and pleasurable erogenous zones with our partners. Similarly, as adults, we can learn safe, respectful ways to engage in anal play in order to add pleasure, intimacy, and variety to our sex lives. As with any other activity, some health risks are involved—but once you know the facts, you can be smart about how you play. Anal sex has been misunderstood for way too long, so it's time to toss out the misconceptions and celebrate the truths. Here are the top ten nasty rumors that have given anal play a bad name:

1. Anal sex is unnatural.
2. Anal sex is dirty and messy.
3. It's painful!
4. It's dangerous.
5. It causes hemorrhoids.
6. I hate rectal exams at the doctor, so I know I won't like anal sex.
7. Anal sex makes men gay.
8. Real men don't have anal sex.
9. Having regular anal sex "loosens" the anus, and I don't want to end up wearing adult diapers!
10. There's simply no such thing as anal pleasure; anal play can't be anything but painful.

Newsflash: None of these statements are true. But if you agreed with some of them, you're not alone. Lots of people aren't acquainted with the realities of adult anal play. That's why it's time to chuck these rumors out the window. Let's get going!

Myth 1:
ANAL SEX IS UNNATURAL

Oh yeah? Well, who decided to put all of the nerve endings there, then, if not for the possibility of pleasure? (And what's more, how "natural" are the rituals and accessories that accompany sex in Western culture—like colored condoms, roses in February, and lacy lingerie?) If the definition of *natural sex* is "penis in vagina for procreation only," then it's safe to say that the vast majority of people aren't following that plan. That's because, for most of us, these parameters are limiting and boring and may not even be possible. Ultimately, the most "natural" sex act is one in which all participants—whether that's one, two, or more—are free to be themselves, to communicate their desires, and to enjoy consensual pleasure without shame. And that may or may not include anal sex. The truth is, anal play is a perfectly natural way for humans to express their sexuality and to give and receive pleasure.

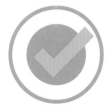

Fact

Anal sex isn't a new phenomenon, and it wasn't "invented" by gay men. People of all genders, sexes, and orientations have been enjoying anal play for thousands of years. In fact, anal penetration has even been observed in polecats, giraffes, and bison, according to Joan Roughgarden in *Evolution's Rainbow: Diversity, Gender, and Sexuality in Nature and People* (2004).

FROM OUR SURVEY

" Pleasure rules. If something feels good and is being explored and enjoyed by consenting adults, then there is absolutely nothing wrong with that. All genders have anuses, which come with sensitive nerve endings that love to receive attention. Sex, in general, is messy. It deals with varying body fluids and inserting body parts inside other body parts. And it is immensely pleasurable and satisfying. Anal doesn't have to be any messier than any other sex act. It's all in the preparation, the readiness, and the timing of the individuals involved. "

Myth 2:
ANAL SEX IS DIRTY AND MESSY

Yes, it can be—but so can cooking, working out, making art, and having just about any kind of uninhibited fun. Anal play isn't necessarily messier than any other type of sex. Regardless of where you're putting what, when we lubricate, ejaculate, add massage oil, use toys, and let our imaginations run wild, we end up with sexy juices and other liquids to wash off or remove afterward. That's fine; it's part of the experience. Anal sex is no different, but enemas, condoms, towels, and baby wipes can help minimize messiness and make cleanup relatively effortless.

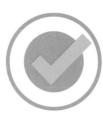

Fact
Anal sex is practiced by neat freaks around the world. With the right tools, you'll be able to enjoy plenty of pleasure without worrying about the consequences.

Myth 3:
ANAL SEX IS PAINFUL

Lots of people—even experienced anal-sex enthusiasts—feel pain at some point during anal sex and assume that pain is simply part of the package. Not so! In fact, pain is often an indication that you're doing something wrong and should change your tactics. For instance, you might be going too fast, you may need to use more lube, or you could be poking the sensitive lining of the rectum. Following some of the advice in the coming chapters can make anal sex fully pleasurable and painless.

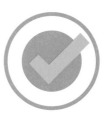

Fact
Anal sex can be delicious and can easily be enjoyed pain-free. (I'll show you how! Chapter 5 will give you all the details.)

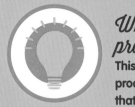

What's a prostate?

This gland produces fluids that mix with sperm in ejaculate. You can feel it through the front of the rectal wall in men and trans women. Stimulating it can provide immense pleasure. It is also an area that is susceptible to growths and cancer. For more about the prostate, see chapter 2.

Myth 4:
ANAL SEX IS DANGEROUS

Well, there are dangers inherent in any kind of sex—and in just about any activity at all, including walking down the street. Many of the dangers of anal sex have been exaggerated, thanks to the negative messages about anal play that run rampant in Western culture. That means it can be tough to tell the difference between reasonable precautions and myths based on fear or ignorance. So plenty of folks who are interested in backdoor play are put off by the idea of tearing sensitive anal tissue, contracting vaginal or urinary-tract infections, ingesting fecal matter, contracting HIV or AIDS, or taking a trip to the emergency room to remove a sex toy that's gotten lost. And that's a shame since there are plenty of ways to prevent all of these concerns. Check out chapter 7 to find out how.

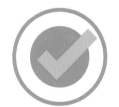

Fact

Safe, healthy anal pleasure is totally possible. It's best when you know and trust your partner, if you're patient and willing to go slowly at first, and when you use anal-specific toys and safer-sex supplies properly. Of course, if you have any medical conditions that affect your digestive tract, prostate, or any other part of your body that you plan to involve in anal sex, be sure to follow the advice your doctor has given you.

Myth 5:
ANAL SEX CAUSES HEMORRHOIDS

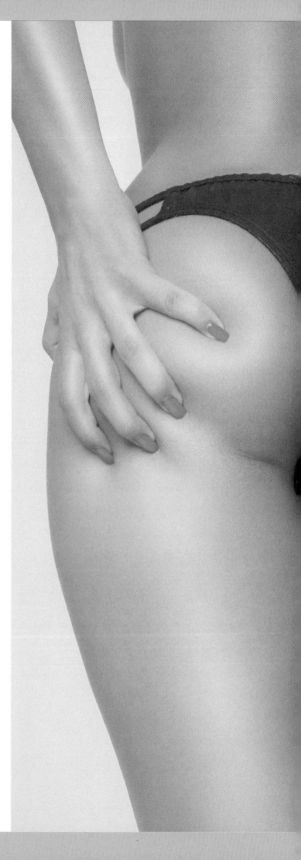

Not necessarily. Hemorrhoids are swollen blood vessels that are located either inside the anus or just outside its opening. For some people, simply sitting, passing a bowel movement, or touching the anal area can be very painful; for others, hemorrhoids aren't painful at all. They result from an increase in pressure in the anal/rectal area caused by any number of things, including holding in a bowel movement or pushing one out, lack of regular exercise, low-fiber diets, pregnancy, or sitting for long periods of time. While it is possible for anal sex to trigger hemorrhoids if the receptive partner strains during the encounter, many anal aficionados believe that slow anal stimulation while the anus is relaxed may even *prevent* hemorrhoids. However, if you have them already and they're painful, it may be worthwhile to avoid anal play until they disappear.

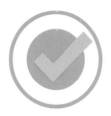

Fact

As long as you take your time and make sure the anus is relaxed before and during penetration, it's unlikely that anal sex will cause hemorrhoids.

FROM OUR SURVEY

" *I do get hemorrhoids, but they've been much better since I started having very regular anal sex.* "

" *The key is to listen to the hemorrhoids, because they will talk to you—scream at you—if you try to ignore them. So you'd be wise to listen and let them take the lead. I prepare myself for anal play, and if my hemorrhoids are active, I don't insert toys or penises. I simply enjoy other anal pleasures, such as oral play.* "

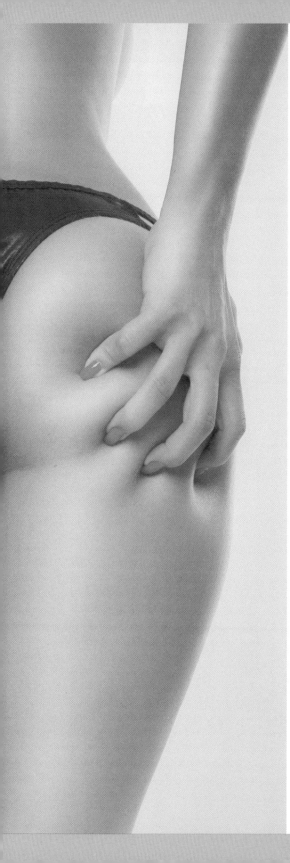

Myth 6:

I SURE AS HECK DIDN'T ENJOY MY LAST RECTAL EXAM, SO I KNOW I WON'T ENJOY ANAL SEX

It's a regular and necessary test for many of us, especially for those of us with prostates—but few people fantasize about rectal exams, in which a doctor checks the prostate and rectum with gloved fingers. And there's a good reason for that. First of all, keep in mind that because your doctor is a medical professional, he or she is not trying to turn you on before entering you.

Au contraire! If your doctor were to touch you the way a lover might, he or she would certainly be slapped with a lawsuit—and fast! But of course this also means that anal penetration as part of a doctor's examination is much more likely to feel painful. Plus, for most of us, a doctor's office is hardly the sexiest location in the world (unless it works for you in your fantasy life!).

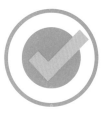

Fact

Most of us don't enjoy rectal exams—even folks who engage in relaxed, hot, sexy anal play in their personal lives.

Myth 7:
ANAL SEX MAKES MEN GAY

I can guarantee you this: having anal sex will not change a person's sexual orientation. That's impossible since each individual person dictates her or his own sexual orientation. Yes, some gay or bisexual men do engage in anal sex, but not all of them. (In case you're wondering what the rest of them are doing, oral sex, fun toys, and kink are all alternative options!) Many men who identify themselves as straight also enjoy receiving anal play because they, too, have an abundance of pleasure-giving nerve endings at the anal opening and at the prostate. The truth is, anal sex is no more gay than kissing is. Anyone can enjoy it, and many straight men get really turned on by the idea of being penetrated by their female partners. And believe me, there's no shortage of women who get turned on by the very same idea—so straight men certainly don't need to change their orientation to enjoy anal play!

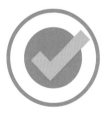

Fact
Some gay and bisexual men enjoy anal play, and some don't. Some straight men enjoy anal play, and some don't. It's as simple as that.

FROM OUR SURVEY

"When I was young, three of my male buddies and I found one of our moms' paperback copies of the then-current The Sensuous Woman and The Joy of Sex and came up with the collective idea of practicing oral and anal sex on each other using tips and techniques from the books. We developed the clumsy but brutally effective technique of coating the cock in petroleum jelly and pushing into the ass with one or two forceful strokes. The first time I entered my friend in this way, it was a feeling of such overwhelming pleasure I knew that I would be chasing sexual bliss for the rest of my life. He squirmed beneath me in discomfort, which only made it feel even better for me. For the next couple of weeks, when it was my turn to bottom, it felt like an unpleasant tradeoff for the chance to experience the pleasure of topping.

But eventually I started to notice that the initial burning discomfort that followed intromission eventually turned into a warm, tickly feeling that radiated out from my ass, into my cock and balls, forward into my belly, and down the backs of my legs to my toes. I was hooked, and being the butt-sex bottom became my favorite part of these sessions."

Myth 8:
REAL MEN DON'T ENGAGE IN ANAL SEX

The so-called rules that govern—or try to govern—what "real" men do (or don't do) limit all of us, regardless of our genders. From the time we're born, we hear certain refrains again and again, and they constrain us throughout our lives. Real men don't cry. Real men don't show emotion. They shouldn't be vulnerable or "act like women" (whatever that means). Within the context of sex, then, the act of being penetrated is sometimes seen as feminine, weak, or submissive. Thus, the story goes, men who "behave like women" sexually are also feminine, weak, or submissive. These stereotypes are untrue, and they disrespect of people of all genders. There is nothing inherently feminine or weak about being penetrated, and—regardless of gender and sexuality—people who allow themselves to be vulnerable and to express their desires are very strong indeed.

I've met such a wide range of people who enjoy being penetrated, and I can assure you that it's got nothing to do with gender, sexuality, skin color, age, profession, or anything else. The equal-opportunity orifice allows everyone to enjoy pleasure—however they want and with whomever they want. And the good news is that people of all genders are working hard to counteract harmful stereotypes about "real" men and to help men and those around them to live authentic, holistic lives.

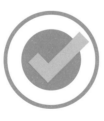

Fact
Real men enjoy whatever brings them (and their partner or partners) true pleasure.

FROM OUR SURVEY

As a trans-feminine, male-bodied person, anal sex is actually an important part of me 'doing' femininity, or having it done to me, I suppose. Anal sex addresses, partially and momentarily, my body dysphoria and helps me to be fucked in ways that feel better for me than being 'the penetrative man.' It allows me to be sexually expressive and responsive in ways that have me be the desired object rather than the desiring subject.

Myth 9:

ANAL SEX "LOOSENS" THE ANUS, AND YOU'LL END UP WEARING ADULT DIAPERS AS A RESULT

This is a really common misconception. Lots of people are afraid that inserting penises or toys into the anus will stretch the muscles irreversibly—as if the anus were made of a type of elastic that can "get tired," so to speak, and won't return to its original shape. (This myth isn't unlike the one you heard in high school about women becoming "loose"—both literally and figuratively—as a result of "too much" sex.) Not at all! The anus doesn't stretch to release a bowel movement or to allow a penis, finger, or toy inside. Instead, the sphincter muscles actually relax in order to accommodate objects passing through. You know the terms *anal-retentive* or *tight-ass*, which describe a person who is so inflexible and tense that he or she holds it all in? This is not the ideal we want to strive for—and it won't help you enjoy anal play, either! As with all muscles, though, warming them up before exercising them is the best way to play.

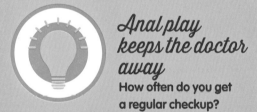

Anal play keeps the doctor away

How often do you get a regular checkup? I bet it's once a year at most. But if you have a prostate, it needs to be monitored for any unwanted (i.e., cancerous) growths. Wouldn't it be great to notice any changes in your prostate as soon as possible? Regular prostate play can help you tune in to subtle changes in sensation—and that'll allow you to get any necessary medical attention much more quickly. For more about the prostate, see chapter 2.

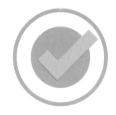

Fact
Plenty of anal-pleasure fans are walking the streets diaper-free as we speak—and you can be one of them, too!

Myth 10:
ANAL PLEASURE IS AN OXYMORON: IT JUST ISN'T POSSIBLE

FROM OUR SURVEY

" *For me, anal orgasms have happened without ejaculation. They are more of a whole-body feeling and don't have a refractory period in the same way that orgasms with ejaculation do. I really like the feeling of them, because they engage the nerves of your entire body and similarly make your entire body feel relaxed afterward, whereas penile orgasms are mostly centered on the penis itself.* "

Think again! Anal play can be intensely enjoyable. So just in case I haven't convinced you yet, it's time to extol the virtues of anal pleasure in detail. Physiologically, backdoor love is very real. The vast number of nerve endings in the anus and perineal sponge or prostate (depending upon your sex) offer the possibility of immense gratification—but how you get there is completely up to you. Some people like external stimulation, while others like to take the plunge and enjoy being penetrated. Some folks combine it with other types of pleasure; others prefer to keep their anal adventures separate from other types of sex play. Lots of anal enthusiasts like thrusting, but others prefer vibration or the sensation of a butt plug that's simply left in place. Some rear-enders just appreciate the pleasurable sensations of anal stimulation; others—of all genders—can orgasm from anal sex. In fact, these orgasms can be incredibly intense. Folks have described the orgasms from anal sex as "hot" and "explosive." If you have a prostate, you're especially lucky, because orgasms from prostate play don't just rock the pelvic area—they seem to ripple throughout the entire body.

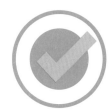

Fact
Anal play can feel great and, like all forms of pleasurable, consensual sex, can actually be good for you. If you'd like to relax the anal area before you get going, pleasure in and around the rosebud (anus) can help. If the rosebud tenses up, slow down or stop the stimulation. Just like a full-body massage, most people prefer slow movements to very fast ones.

Chapter 2

YOUR ANAL ANATOMY:
MEET THE EQUAL-OPPORTUNITY ORIFICE

Although we tend to focus on our differences as humans, our bodies are pretty similar to each other's. Sure, we might have varying sexual experiences depending on what's between our legs, but like kissing, anal sex—especially with shallow penetration—pretty much feels the same for everyone. Sex-dependent differences in anal anatomy become a factor once you get further than 1 inch (2.5 cm) inside, but the anus itself is truly an equal-opportunity orifice: almost everybody has one!

To fully enjoy anal pleasure, it's helpful to know how your backdoor anatomy works. There's no harm in knowing a little more about what else goes on back there. Most of us don't like to talk about the (very necessary!) bodily functions that take place at the rear of the bus, but they're part of life—and understanding them can help you enjoy and relax into anal pleasure a bit more. After all, knowledge is power!

So get ready for a crash course in anal anatomy. This chapter will show you everything you need to know. You'll learn about your erogenous zones and exactly what happens when you get aroused. You'll find out why knowing all about pooping is a good thing, and you'll be able to start exploring your anal area gently and mindfully.

First things first: Here's a handy rundown of your anal anatomy—what it's called, what it looks like, and what it's for.

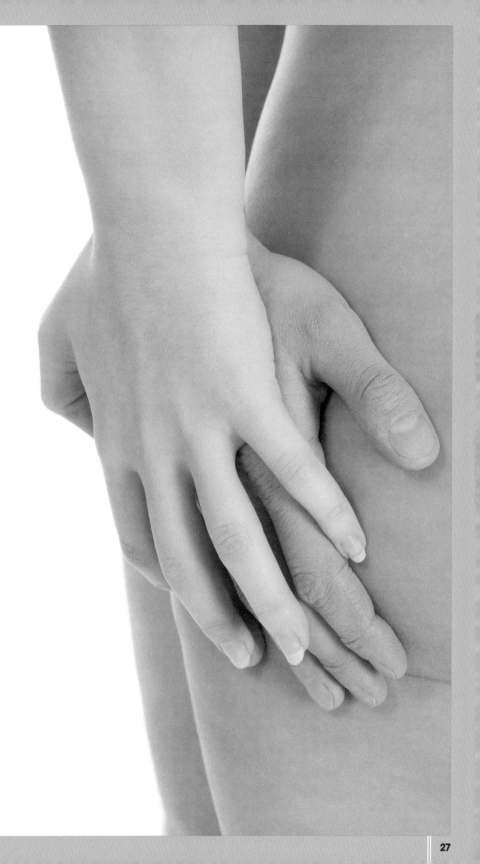

ANAL ANATOMY

Male/Outie

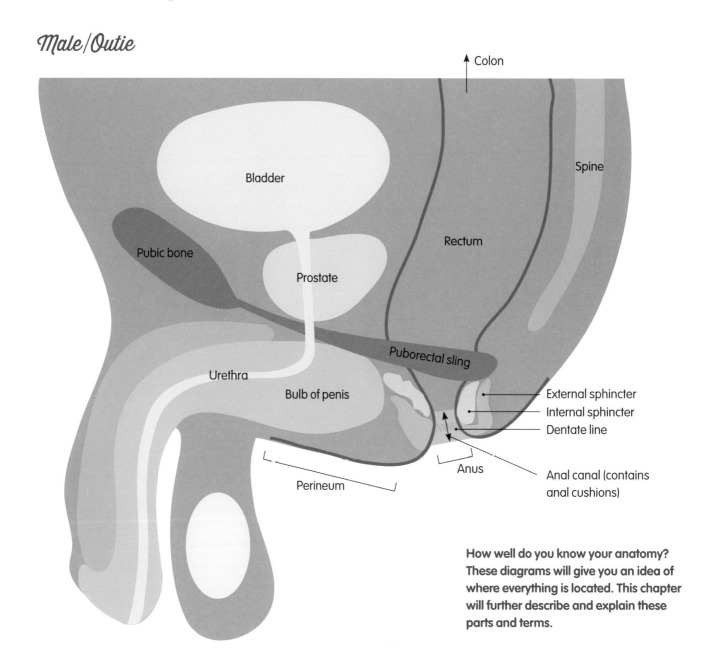

Colon

Bladder

Spine

Pubic bone

Rectum

Prostate

Puborectal sling

Urethra

Bulb of penis

External sphincter

Internal sphincter

Dentate line

Anus

Anal canal (contains anal cushions)

Perineum

How well do you know your anatomy? These diagrams will give you an idea of where everything is located. This chapter will further describe and explain these parts and terms.

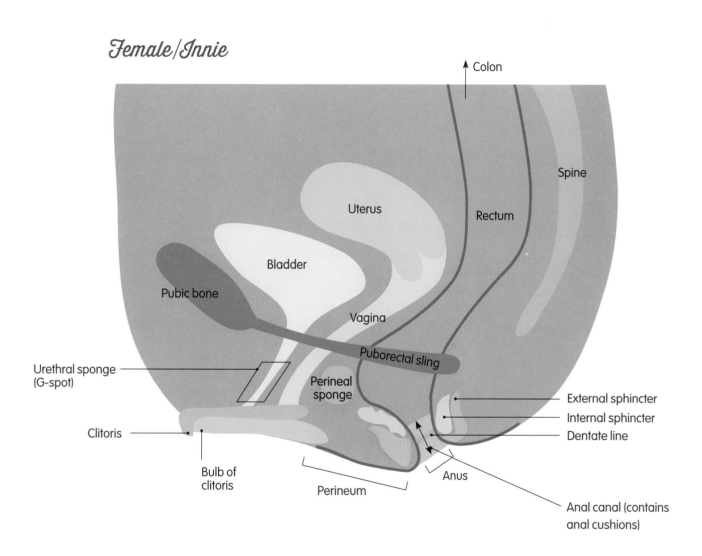

Female/Innie

Colon

Spine

Uterus

Rectum

Bladder

Pubic bone

Vagina

Puborectal sling

Urethral sponge
(G-spot)

Perineal
sponge

External sphincter

Internal sphincter

Dentate line

Clitoris

Bulb of
clitoris

Perineum

Anus

Anal canal (contains
anal cushions)

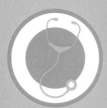

Respect your sphincters

The anal sphincters contribute the most to fecal continence. If they are overstretched, punctured, or torn, their function may become impaired, resulting in fecal incontinence (not being able to hold in your bowel movements, or BMs). There is no effective surgical repair for such damage. Pay attention to your body while playing!

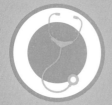

Be careful what you insert!

Anal play with an object without a flared base can be extremely dangerous. Anyone who has worked in an emergency department of a hospital knows the myriad of items that get lodged in people's butts. And it is not always possible to retrieve these objects easily from the rectum. In extreme cases, patients have required laparotomies to remove such items, which involves a large incision through the abdominal wall to gain access. The bowels and digestive tract rarely function the same after such surgery, and fecal incontinence is often a result.

FROM OUR SURVEY

" Hemorrhoids. They hurt! Going slow, using lots of lube, being fully relaxed, and being turned on first—having had at least one orgasm—helps to prevent blood vessels from tearing and hemorrhoids from occurring or getting in the way. "

Anus

The anus is made of folds of soft tissue that can expand, giving it its puckered look, similar to fabric-covered hairbands or scrunchies that bunch up when not stretched taut. The anus itself is filled with many blood vessels and tons of nerve endings, and it's often a different color from the skin around it, just like your genitals are. The area surrounding the anus contains hair follicles, although actual hair may or may not be visible. Some folks have hair like peach fuzz that can be felt but not seen, while others have dark, thick hair that's easy to spot—and there are countless variations in between. My first anal teacher, Chester, called the anus "the rosebud." It sounds a little friendlier and less medical.

Anal canal

The end of the large intestine, this opening becomes engorged with blood during arousal and expands when relaxed, allowing things to pass through. It extends approximately 1½ inches (3.8 cm) inward, but most of the pleasure it produces is felt in the first third of it, below what is called the dentate line. Below the dentate line, the anal canal's sensitivity is similar to that of outer skin and is sensitive to pain, pleasure, and temperature. Above the dentate line, in the inner two-thirds of the canal, the tissue is sensitive to stretching sensations only.

Anal sphincters

Your anal canal comes equipped with two anal sphincter muscles, with the external sphincter surrounding the internal one. As you insert a finger, you'll feel the external then the internal sphincter muscles. The external sphincter is under your conscious control. When you squeeze your anus tightly to stop a bowel movement (BM), you're squeezing the external sphincter. The movement of the internal sphincter, on the other hand, is involuntary. Your body controls it in the same way it controls your heart rate and circulation. It tenses when you feel fear or anxiety. These two sphincters can expand when relaxed, which is why it is important to stay relaxed whenever your anus is involved—during anal play or when passing BMs. Your sphincters act a little like a drawstring. With tension, the drawstring is pulled and the hole becomes smaller, making it hard to pass anything comfortably through the middle. But they can also relax significantly. In fact, under anesthesia, these muscles can relax enough to accommodate a doctor's hand— for example, in the unfortunate event that something inappropriate for anal play was inserted and cannot be pushed out on its own.

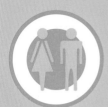

What's an outie?

An *outie* is another name for a penis. A vulva/vagina can be called an *innie*. We call our body parts by many different names, some with positive connotations and others with negative connotations. Trans people in particular, who often feel like they were born in the wrong body, may not like to call their genitals by their clinical or standard names. A trans woman, for example, may not like to label her genitals a penis because of its masculine connotation. She may call it her clit instead. Or she may like to call it an outie, which has no associations other than belly buttons, which are pretty innocuous. In this book, I will occasionally use the words *outie* or *innie* to use language inclusive for those who do not like to refer to their body parts as penises or vulvas/vaginas. Thanks to the youth at Planned Parenthood Toronto who suggested these terms at a workshop I held!

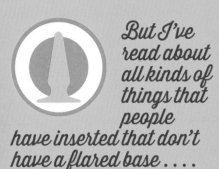

But I've read about all kinds of things that people have inserted that don't have a flared base . . . .

Well, I am sure you have read all sorts of things online that are likely not great ideas to imitate in real life. Some people may have been lucky to get away with a risky toy one, five, or even a hundred times. But eventually they may not be so lucky and may find themselves at the emergency ward. There's a reason there's a popular television show about being sent to the hospital after sex—things often go wrong when you don't take proper precautions. Better to be safe than eventually sorry!

Rectum

The rectum is a mucous membrane that acts as a passageway extending about 5–6 inches (12.7–15.2 cm) past the anal opening, and it doesn't normally store feces in people with healthy bowel movements. That's because healthy BMs—that is, "Goldilocks" BMs that are neither too hard nor too soft—tend to leave next to nothing behind on their exit. (There may be traces of poop left behind after your last BM, but otherwise, the rectum shouldn't contain any fecal matter.) The rectum is lined with rectal fluid, mucus designed to trap bacteria and viruses and protect the rectum. The mucus also serves as a gentle lubricant to allow smooth passage of BMs. The nerves of the rectum are less sensitive than those of the anus and anal canal, and that means that it registers pressure more easily than it can discern between various types of touch. The rectum is also much roomier and can expand more easily than the anus—which is why a finger, penis, or toy can move more freely once it's more than 1 inch (2.5 cm) inside. But there is a downside to that extra space. Once something without a flared base is inserted, it's really hard to get it out. (Moral of the story: Never put anything inside your anus unless it has a flared base!) Also, the rectum is not a straight line; it's shaped more like an *S*, angling forward and then backward. The rectum also absorbs water from BMs, which means that it'll also absorb lubricant or any other fluids you insert into it. Always read the ingredients listed on your lube's label!

Anal cushions

Anal cushions are three prominent vertical "columns" that lie below the surface of the anal canal. They're not unlike the penis in the sense that they at times are engorged with blood and at other times are not. They fill with blood to keep the anus closed most of the time and to assist with continence (holding in poop). Blood drains from them before you pass a bowel movement or when the anal sphincters relax during anal play. They may become displaced when you strain to have a BM, and they are vulnerable to trauma and bleed readily when damaged. So be nice to your anal cushions!

FROM OUR SURVEY

" I do have hemorrhoids, but I find getting slowly, gently fingered before sex helps put things where they should be. Aggressive sex afterward sometimes makes them worse later, but it's worth it. "

Puborectal sling, or puborectalis muscle

This muscle is the first gateway for controlling or stopping a BM or gas. It's literally "slung" around the rectum as if it were a scarf or rope wrapped around a person's waist and held tightly in place. If you're holding the scarf and you pull it toward you, the other person has to bend in accordance with the tension. In the same way, the tighter the muscle, the tighter the curve of the rectum. When the muscle relaxes, the rectum straightens out, making it easier for BMs, penises, or toys to pass in or out. But if you're not relaxed, the tense muscles will bend the rectum sharply, making it more challenging and less pleasurable for things to pass in or out of the rectum.

Colon

The sigmoid colon is located just past the rectum on the way up your large intestine. It's about 7 inches (17.8 cm) inside, so unless you're playing with a very long penis or toy, you probably won't get up that far. And that's not entirely a bad thing, since this is the area where poop is stored. When enough waste material accumulates and the pressure in the colon builds, the colorectal sphincter releases and the bowel movement makes its way down through the rectum and out the anus. Those who like deep penetration, take note. The colorectal sphincter can be hard to get past.

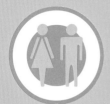

What are hemorrhoids?

When we don't relax—whether that's a result of daily stress, straining to have a bowel movement, or tensing up during anal play—blood doesn't drain from the anal cushions, and that can cause them to become distended or misshapen. With frequent distension, the anal cushion stretches and creates a hemorrhoid. Internal hemorrhoids occur above the dentate line. They do not usually feel painful because we don't have pain receptors in that area, but they may leave evidence of their existence in the form of red blood on toilet paper, toys, or body parts. Sometimes they protrude to the outside, which is often quite painful. External hemorrhoids occur below the dentate line and are usually painful because of the sensitive nerve endings in that region.

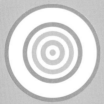

Comfortable penetration

Get into the fetal position or any other position in which your legs are at a right angle or closer to your body. Positions like these straighten out your rectum. This way, whatever you're putting inside won't have to navigate the same acute twists and turns in its journey as it would if your body were lying straight with your rectum curved.

" Awesome, body-quivering, mind-blowing. [My prostate orgasms] are without ejaculation. Very different, as you don't just stop like you do after a normal orgasm. . . . With a prostate orgasm, you just want more of it, and you keep on going. With P-play, once you're aroused, you get so into it. "

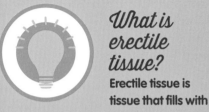

What is erectile tissue?

Erectile tissue is tissue that fills with blood when you're sexually aroused. The parts of your body that sport erectile tissue are erogenous zones, and touching them usually feels good. In general, the more engorged with blood the area is, the better it feels when it's touched. Erectile tissue can be found in the following areas:

1. Clitoris

2. Vestibular bulbs (located under the surface of the skin and just under and outside the inner labia)

3. G-spot or urethral sponge, which surrounds the urethra and can be felt on the front wall of the vagina

4. Perineal sponge, or P-spot, which is located on the back wall of the vagina, between the vagina and the anus

5. Penis

(And guess what: There's also a little bit of erectile tissue at the opening to the nose!)

NON-ANAL EROGENOUS ZONES

Of course, your anus isn't the only sensitive spot in your genital area. Experiment with these hot spots, too.

Perineum

This area is also known as the 'taint—as in, "it ain't the testicles, and 't ain't the butthole, either." In men, it's sometimes called the manbridge. The perineum lies between the anus and either the vagina or the testicles, depending on which set of equipment you own. From here, the base of the penis or the perineal sponge can be stimulated, which some folks find incredibly arousing. While it's possible to stimulate the prostate indirectly from the perineum, it's not a terribly effective access point for the prostate.

Perineal sponge

This little-known nub of erectile tissue is located between the vagina and the anus, about a thumb's depth (1–2 inches [2.5–5 cm]) inside. It engorges with blood during arousal, and some folks find stimulating it to be wonderfully pleasurable. Not everyone is a fan, but it's well worth experimenting to see whether it works for you and/or your partner! It can be stimulated through the posterior, or back, vaginal wall; the anterior, or front, anal wall; or both ways at the same time. Some people like the sensation of a single finger on one or both sides of the perineal sponge; others enjoy the feeling of a finger on one side and a penis or toy on the other. Still others like toys and/or penises on either side. The combinations are endless!

Pelvic floor muscles

These infamous muscles are usually discussed within the context of post-childbirth recovery, but the fact is, people of all genders and sexes need to keep them in good shape in order to maintain urinary continence and pelvic floor health. They're a network of muscles that support all of your internal organs, so it's important to keep them strong. (Plus, healthy muscles also help keep your nerves alert. That's vital, since nerves are responsible for delivering neurological impulses—such as pleasure!—to the brain.) Pelvic floor muscles contract at random during arousal and contract rhythmically at 1 second intervals during orgasm. If you're not sure where these muscles are, try this: Next time you're peeing, squeeze the muscles you use to stop the flow of urine. Those are your pelvic floor muscles, and you need to exercise them. Don't stop the flow of urine every time you use the bathroom; doing so is bad for your bladder. Instead, try to do up to two hundred squeezes throughout each day. Squeeze for 5 seconds, and then relax for 5 seconds. If you like, you can squeeze against a finger, a toy, or something specifically designed for pelvic floor exercises, also known as Kegels. You can do them while you're having sex, or when you're driving, reading, or doing the dishes. Talk about multitasking!

Prostate

The prostate has gotten a lot of airtime recently, thanks to its association with prostate cancer prevention efforts and the Movember Foundation. But it's equally well-known in some circles for the pleasure possibilities it offers. Yessir, people with penises have more to celebrate than just their cocks and testicles. They've also got prostates, which some folks would argue can provide the most intense pleasure of all. This famous gland isn't located in the rectum, but you can feel it easily through the anterior (front) wall of the rectum, around 2–4 inches (5–10 cm) inside. It surrounds the urethra like a donut, and it swells with fluid during arousal, which makes it bulge toward the rectal wall. (The fluid produced by the prostate accounts for about one-third of the ejaculate that mixes with sperm so that they can flow freely to their destination.) This swelling makes it easier and more pleasurable to feel during arousal, or even just before ejaculation. In general, most men or trans women will be immediately aware of their prostates once they're stimulated. (If not, then it's likely when they're even more aroused.) An exploratory finger will often feel a dip and then a bulge around the prostate—like a small island with a moat around it. It feels a little like a 2-inch (5-cm) tomato, firm but yielding a bit when pressed.

G-spot

This often-elusive erogenous zone can be felt through the anterior, or front, wall of the vagina, just as the prostate can be felt through the anterior wall of the rectum. Some people with sensitive G-spots report that they can feel this area during anal stimulation, all the way through both the rectal and vaginal walls, while others have trouble locating it even just vaginally. If you fall it into the latter category, you might find it easier to try to stimulate your perineal sponge during anal play.

Bulb of clitoris or penis

The base of the clitoris and vestibular bulbs and the base of the penis are both anterior to (in front of) the rectum. When fully aroused, some people can stimulate these areas through shallow penetration of the anus and rectum, angling toward the belly button—but most people probably won't find the sensations very intense.

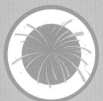

Do your pelvic floor squeezes

You know pelvic floor squeezes are important for your health—but did you know that strong pelvic floor muscles can also intensify sexual pleasure and orgasm? Try your squeezes during solo or partner sex. It'll feel fabulous since your erectile tissues are sandwiched right between those muscles. It's also a great way to get over the hump when you're close to orgasm; a few well-timed squeezes can push you right over the edge. And, of course, you can also do pelvic floor exercises when you're not having sex—either way, they'll strengthen your muscles, which means you'll have better orgasms and fewer health problems. People with weak pelvic floor muscles tend to experience incontinence or, in more serious cases, prolapse of the bladder through the wall of the vagina. That can be incredibly painful and can even require surgery. So keep squeezing!

FROM OUR SURVEY

" I've noticed a big difference in my orgasms since I started doing my Kegels. I love that I can orgasm from internal sex now—and that I can squirt! "

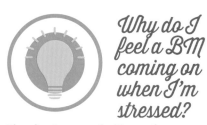

Why do I feel a BM coming on when I'm stressed?

The short answer is, it's another articulation of the fight-or-flight response. Your body is hardwired to react this way when it senses danger—say, if there's a bear chasing you. When you feel stressed or anxious, your body snaps into fight-or-flight mode. Norepinephrine, adrenaline, and cortisol hormones are released, and blood sugar floods the body to provide you with extra energy so you can either fight hard or run fast. Blood flows away from the genital area (it's not a good time to have sex when a bear is on your tail), your digestion slows down, and the bowels empty so that you'll be carrying less weight. Our bodies think of everything, don't they?

A BRIEF DIGRESSION ON POOP

To quote the infamous children's book of the same name, everybody poops. If you're going to enjoy anal pleasure, you need to be down with it. Why? Because—along with the possibility of pleasure—that's what your anal anatomy is there for. Here's a quick rundown on how the pooping process works.

When you eat, your muscles move the material through the 30 feet (9 m) of your digestive tract using a wavelike process called peristalsis (similar to how an earthworm moves). After your body has absorbed the nutrients and goodness from the food, the leftover waste needs to be eliminated. Between one and four times a day in most people, often after waking up or eating, the gastrocolic reflex pushes waste toward the rectum. When the colon is filled with waste, that waste places pressure on the colorectal sphincter to signal that the gates need to open because a BM is on its way down (and that, handily enough, gives you time to find a bathroom). Blood drains from your anal cushions. Then, as pressure in the rectum rises, the defecation reflex is triggered, the internal sphincter and puborectalis muscle relax, and contractions push the poop out.

Whether you're engaging in anal play or not, it's healthiest to let your BM pass as soon as you feel the urge (if a bathroom is nearby, of course). If you don't, your rectum absorbs some of the liquid in the stool, making it harder to pass. And the more you ignore the rectal reflex, the lazier it becomes. That means you might have to strain to pass a BM, increasing the possibility of developing hemorrhoids. It's also more likely that bits of fecal matter will be left behind in the rectum after a BM, something most people try to avoid when they pursue anal pleasure. Finally, repeated restraint of BMs can result in tense pelvic muscles. Tense muscles are not really desirable anywhere, but in the pelvic floor they can lead to pain and more straining to pass a BM.

What's normal when it comes to poop? "Normal" varies from person to person, and most medical professionals agree that going anywhere between three times per day and three times per week is pretty regular and healthy. Of course, if your stools are too hard or too soft or if you strain to pass a BM, then it's probably a good idea to change your diet and personal habits to help you have healthier poops. Getting plenty of exercise, enjoying a high-fiber diet, drinking lots of non-caffeinated fluids, listening to your body when it tells you to find a bathroom, and eating regular meals will help keep things running smoothly.

And when it comes to anal play, it's important to tune in to your own version of "normal." Some folks suggest using the toilet before engaging in anal play—but most of us can't just have a BM on demand. That's why it's a good idea to get a sense of your individual internal rhythm if you want to play with your butt. Knowing that a BM is not in your near future will help you to relax and enjoy the experience. For instance, if you're a one-a-day kind of person and you haven't had your daily BM yet, and you happen to feel frisky at, say, 8 p.m., then perhaps today is not the best

day for anal play. Not only are you more likely to have a BM while you're playing (especially if you're feeling stressed), you'll also be focusing on that BM and whether it's on the way. That's not going to help you relax into the pleasure. Similarly, if you're a one-a-day kind of person, you had a BM during the day, and you've stuck to a regular routine (no spicy foods or sudden stress), you can probably feel pretty confident that the anal sensations you're experiencing during anal play are a result of pleasure rather than signals that a BM is on its way. You'll be much more likely to relax and simply enjoy all of the information that your nerve endings are telling you about what is going on in there.

If the idea of butt play makes you feel stressed, you may be bringing on the very BM you're trying to avoid. So take some deep breaths and remind yourself that you're not in any danger and that you get to decide how far—and whether—you want to proceed.

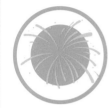

Straighten out your rectum

Our bodies are designed to squat while emptying our bowels. The squatting position allows the rectum to straighten out and lets gravity assist in the process of evacuation. Toilets are a relatively modern invention, and when you sit on one, your rectum remains in its relative *S* shape, making BMs slightly more challenging to pass. Most of us with healthy BMs don't notice the difference. However, if passing BMs is not easy for you, then try pulling your knees to your chest by leaning forward or sitting up, resting your feet on something almost as tall as the toilet, bringing your legs up to your chest and resting your spine against the back of the toilet, or even squatting on the toilet. When trying any of these positions, make sure you have something sturdy to balance on safely so that you don't fall! The gravity and angle of being upright in the squatting position can be much healthier for safe and comfortable passage.

THE MECHANICS OF AROUSAL

Before we took a detour into your digestive tract, we were talking about arousal. That's much sexier—so let's head back to the fun stuff!

When you're aroused, blood floods your pelvic region, filling both erectile tissues and anal tissues. (Squeezing the pelvic floor muscles and external sphincter can help some people feel more sensation in these areas.) With anal play, the penis might get hard, stay hard, or lose its erection, so keep in mind that a flaccid penis—especially during prostate play—doesn't necessarily indicate that the possessor of the penis isn't aroused. Some people just find that their arousal shifts its focus to the anal region. Fluid fills and enlarges the prostate or the G-spot to prepare for ejaculation. With ejaculation—which is sometimes, but not always, accompanied by orgasm—the fluid is pushed into the urethra and is then expelled through it.

Post-orgasm, relaxation sets in, and the blood flows away from the erectile tissues, sometimes slowly and sometimes immediately. The anal area also becomes relaxed post-orgasm, and some folks who suffer from pelvic pain find that this relaxation mitigates it and can help them enjoy more pleasure after they come. For these reasons, some folks prefer to engage in butt play after an orgasm so that they're less tense and can fully surrender to the pleasure.

EXPLORING YOUR ANAL ANATOMY: MAKE A DATE WITH YOUR BUTT

Have you made friends with your butt yet? If not, it's time to say hello. Even if you're already enjoying anal play, it can be both powerful and pleasurable to take a step back and revisit the basics. You may discover subtleties and erogenous zones you'd missed during earlier encounters. As you explore, stay aware of your breathing, your emotions, and your thoughts as well as the physical sensations that arise. Anal play can trigger many emotions—positive ones, negative ones, and mixed or ambivalent ones—so sometimes it can be helpful to tune in to the messages in your body and focus on the positive sensations. Then again, sometimes it's better not to dwell on them but to simply notice them and continue mindfully with the experience. Some people like to keep a notebook in which they record their emotions, sensations, and thoughts, especially if they want to remember them to process the experience later with a partner, therapist, coach, or sex-positive friend.

Even if your rational mind tells you otherwise, sometimes anal play can trigger feelings of shame or anxiety. We might have internalized the negative messages surrounding anal play, so our bodies interpret anal play as something that's wrong, dirty, or perverted. These messages often manifest themselves in shallow breathing and tight muscles, so pay attention to the tension in your body, especially in your pelvis. You might also feel that tension in your neck, back, chest, or even your butt. Pay attention to your jaw, because if your anus is tense, your jaw—the opposite end of the digestive tract—will often feel tense as well. Try to relax all of your muscles and breathe deeply, since the fast, shallow breaths that can accompany uncomfortable emotions actually limit levels of sensation. Short, quick breathing defends the body against anticipated or actual pain by restricting what it feels. That's less than ideal for the exercise outlined in this section, because you'll want to progress slowly, without pressure or an agenda, and your goal is to feel as much as you can. Deep breaths will help to relax your body and enable you to sink into the pleasure. Let your tummy rise as your diaphragm fills, and then release your breath slowly and fully. A mantra can be helpful in reversing the negative messages

your body retains and in sending positive thoughts to your brain and body. A typical mantra is often a simple word or phrase like *om* or *peace*, but you can create one that feels authentic to you, such as *I love my butt* or *Pleasure is my choice*. Once you've found one that feels right, repeat the phrase on every outbreath, like a meditation.

During their first few experiences with internal anal play, most people interpret *any* feeling at the back door as a BM. That's because, until you start to experiment with anal play, the only thing going on in your anal area is the expulsion of a BM—so, naturally, the body interprets any sensation there as this familiar event. And, of course, that sensation can cause you to tense up your pelvic region for fear of having a BM during sex. It's a good idea to explore on your own first; that way, you'll become familiar with these sensations without worrying about whether your partner might witness a BM (an unlikely event, but generally an undesirable one). It also allows you to get used to the variety of sensations that can be experienced in the anal area. You'll learn to associate some of these feelings with pleasure and to distinguish the pleasurable sensations from the ones that signal defecation.

You might want to begin your exploration in the shower or bath, which can help you relax and feel "clean" while you explore. Consider giving yourself a manicure since this type of experimentation is generally easier, safer, and more comfortable when you have neatly trimmed fingernails (especially when it comes to internal play). Always take your time. The most exquisite pleasures can be evoked by

the slightest of movements or found in the unlikeliest of places. And you don't have to do everything at once, either. You can choose to explore externally at first and then wait to try penetration.

There's no need to rush the process, so if anything feels painful, stop and try again another day. Seek medical advice if you feel that something is not quite right. Sometimes, though, you might notice that anal play doesn't feel *bad*, just different. In the same way that your anus tenses up the first few times something enters because it feels unfamiliar, your body often sends distress signals when it experiences new sensations. Remember the first time you touched your genitals or your first orgasm (if you can!). Or think about a time you tried a new, challenging physical activity, or even a new food. Our first reactions often contain discomfort, even if that discomfort is mixed with—or overwhelmed by—pleasure. If you proceed too quickly, this "surprise" factor can lead your body to label the new experience as uncomfortable. As you proceed slowly and consciously through this exercise, try to discern the difference between what feels new and what actually feels uncomfortable or painful. Here's how to start. . . .

8 STEPS TO EXPLORING YOUR ANUS

1. Touch your perineum and then contract your pelvic floor muscles. See if you can feel the different muscles move as they tense and release under your fingers. While holding your fingers against your perineum, breathe and release. Notice how your perineum responds.

2. Gradually approach the anus with a finger and notice the difference in sensations as you get closer to your rosebud.

3. Run your finger gently over the folds of and the area around the anus. Notice the difference in sensations and how your body reacts to them. Pay attention to any bulges; become familiar with the landscape. Note your thoughts and emotions, too.

4. Hold your breath and then breathe out. Feel your body's tension level change. Notice the texture of each individual area and how it feels under your finger as you explore.

5. Try different techniques as you experiment. (Chapter 5 has plenty of ideas!) For instance, pull your butt cheeks apart. Play with the doorbell (i.e., push against the anus) and make little and big circles around the anus.

6. Put some lubricant on your finger if you want to explore the anal canal. If you're still in the shower or bath, an oil- or silicone-based lube will stay in place on your finger; the water won't wash it away immediately. If you're out of the water by now, any water-based lube will work, too. Place your finger at your anal opening, squeeze your sphincters, and then relax and allow your finger to slide inside on an outbreath. Don't force it; it may take a few breaths to get to the first knuckle. Pay attention to the subtle sensations that arise. Your instinct may tell you to thrust your finger in and out, but this time, just leave your finger in place.

7. Move your finger in different directions as if your anus were a clock, and figure out which of the twelve "hours" feels best to you. Squeeze your pelvic muscles and sphincter. Notice the sensations that squeezing produces.

8. Play with sensation at various depths. As you explore, notice how different movements create different sensations for your anal canal, your rectum, your finger, and any other part of your body, especially anywhere you naturally store tension. Pay attention to any thoughts or emotions that arise. If you find it helpful, use your mantra. Make a conscious choice to continue exploring or to stop and try again another time.

When you're clean and you've dried yourself off, take a good look at your butt. Squat over a mirror, or lie on your back with your knees bent and hold a magnifying mirror near your knees, angling it so that you can see your beautiful rosebud. It's especially important to do this if you want to enjoy anal exploration with a partner since it'll be easier to relax and let go when you're familiar with your own anatomy. While you're holding the mirror, touch yourself in the same way you did while you were in the bath so that you can watch *and* feel how your body responds. Seeing your body respond to pleasure is an amazing experience, so take the time to enjoy it!

Once you've finished your exploration session, stay aware of your butt for the rest of the day. Notice whether it's tense or relaxed. Do some squeezes to wake it up and say hello. Pay attention also to your whole pelvic region. Note whether your hips feel locked or flexible, whether your pelvic floor is tight or relaxed, and whether your anus is tense or relaxed and open. Mindfulness and meditation are powerful tools for reducing stress and can help you take a grounded approach to everything you do—including anal pleasure. Concentrate on your breathing and scan your whole body, butt included, several times per day. Doing so will encourage you to stay calm, conscious, and aware. That's great for your sex life and your daily life as well!

Now that you're an expert in anal anatomy, it's time to learn how to prep for anal play. Chapter 3 will show you how.

FROM OUR SURVEY

" *I love feeling my body's subtle responses. Sometimes I enjoy just feeling the muscles squeezing and relaxing, [holding] my hand at different places between my vagina and my butthole in the shower, or simply feeling the water run between my butt cheeks.* "

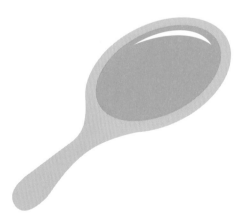

Chapter 3

GETTING READY FOR ANAL PLAY:
PREP, CLEANING, AND SAFETY

You've decided to be adventurous and experiment with anal play for the first time—or for the zillionth time. What do you need to do to prepare yourself? The short answer is nothing at all.

You don't have to do anything special before you play. It's fine to be spontaneous. Nevertheless, many anal enthusiasts like to do certain things to ready themselves, and everyone has individual preferences and routines. For example, some people like to bathe, shower, or clean themselves in other ways before having sex, whether or not anal play is on the table. Others might think about what they've eaten recently—as well as their BM rhythms—before deciding whether now is a good time for anal pleasure. Still others like to clean themselves internally or shave—although that's purely a matter of preference, and it's completely optional.

But there are a few essentials when it comes to prepping for anal sex. It's important to be educated on sexually transmitted infections and to have safer-sex supplies on hand before anal play begins—even if you're in a monogamous relationship. You'll want to have some lube nearby *before* you start. For some folks, not just any lube will do, so be sure you have a supply of your favorite type on hand ahead of time. And of course you'll need to do a little cleanup afterward, so it's good to plan ahead for what you'll need. Again, none of these things are imperative,

but most anal-play aficionados do contemplate at least some of these issues (and discuss them with a partner, if they're enjoying anal with someone else) before sex.

You might want to think about avoiding certain foods beforehand, or you might be curious about pre-sex enemas. And what about shaving and hair removal, or how to make post-sex cleanup as quick and easy as possible? If this all sounds a bit overwhelming, never fear. This chapter will give you the lowdown on how to prep for anal play in the way that's right for you.

A HEALTHY DIET MEANS BETTER ANAL SEX

As a general rule, happy bowel movements make for happier anal-sex experiences. And happier bowel movements happen when your diet is high in fiber, which helps waste move through your digestive tract, leaving only minimal traces of its presence behind. Fruits, vegetables, whole grains, nuts, and legumes are all excellent sources of fiber. (Of course, if you suffer from irritable bowel syndrome [IBS], diarrhea, or other medical conditions, and your health-care provider has suggested that you avoid fiber-rich foods, please heed her or his advice.) Seeds like sesame, chia, and flax are good sources of fiber, too, but they're more likely to be left behind on their way out and could irritate the rectal lining with friction, so think about skipping them if you're planning an anal-play date. The same goes for strawberries, raspberries, and berry jams. Spicy foods can make things move faster and may irritate sensitive tissue, such as the head of the penis of a penetrator or the rectum of the penetratee. Depending on how well your body is accustomed to them, you might want to skip the jalapeños if you're feeling frisky.

But for how long should you abstain from foods like these before anal sex? Think of it like this: It takes 16 to 30 hours for a meal to make its way through your digestive tract, depending on what kind of food you've consumed (e.g., fruits move quickly; fat and meats take longer); how much water you've drunk (staying hydrated promotes good digestion); whether you exercise regularly (exercise speeds up the process); and your age and whether you take certain prescription medications (both of which can slow it down).

Speaking of medication, some over-the-counter remedies can help keep your digestion on an even keel. Metamucil adds extra fiber, speeds digestion, and loosens stools, while Imodium slows things down and firms up loose stools. They're both easy to take—according to your doctor's advice, of course—and can be good for regulating BMs. But prescription medications are another story; some can affect the regularity and consistency of your BMs and might impact pain levels, libido, and sexual response. That's why it's important to take note of your individual responses to your pharmaceuticals and the timing of their effects. That way, you can plan around them and ensure that they interfere as little as possible with your sexual adventures.

"Very important: if your partner likes spicy food, and they've eaten a really spicy meal, wear a condom before you put your cock in their ass, even if you're fluid-bonded. For several years I was in a long-distance relationship, and one time right before my return flight to Toronto, I had anal sex with my lover. Perhaps it was because of all the lube, but I didn't notice at first—though as I started to fuck my lover's ass more and more vigorously, I began to notice this burning sensation. And even after a quick hop in the shower before heading to the airport, it still felt like my cock was on fire for much of the flight home."

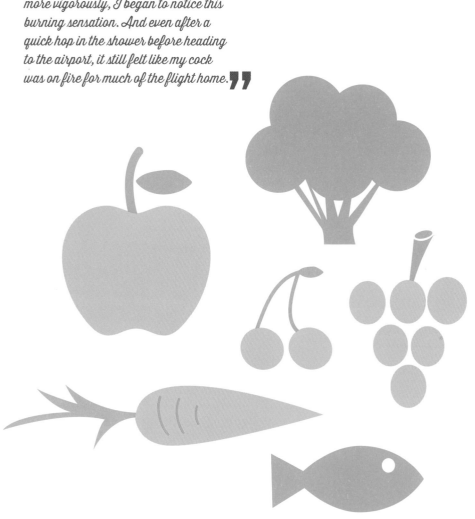

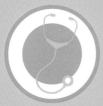

A few thoughts on anal play and IBS

Irritable Bowel Syndrome (IBS) sufferers are used to thinking about every piece of food they eat, but when it comes to anal play, it's not just the food that matters. I have to think about my body's schedule—what it feels like in the morning versus the evening—and consider any adjustments I can make so that playtime is more fun. I tend to stick with easy-to-digest foods ahead of time if there's a chance some anal play might end up happening, and I always forgive myself if there's a little mess. Everyone makes a mess at some point! IBS doesn't have to mean no playtime, though. Once you find out your body's particular rhythm, it's actually pretty easy to incorporate anal play into your sex life (maybe a little more this time, maybe a little less another). I learned early on not to push myself. If something is going to make me feel uncomfortable during or after, I stay away from it; this knowledge comes from experimenting, though. It's nice to reclaim the bum . . . for fun!

—From Samantha Fraser, organizer of the Playground conference

KEEPING IT CLEAN

FROM OUR SURVEY

" *I have not explored much beyond massage, butt plugs, and small dildos and haven't found this level of play to be particularly messy.* "

Externally

Don't worry! Good anal hygiene is easy and basically boils down to common sense. When you were a kid, remember how you were told not to touch your poop and to wash your hands after using the bathroom? The same rules apply to anal sex. Fecal matter can transmit parasites (although they're not as common as most sexually transmitted infections [STIs], it's still a possibility), hepatitis, and E. coli, either through direct oral contact or indirectly via your hands or other intermediaries. So it's a good idea to wash your anal area with regular soap. There's no need to use a heavy-duty industrial soap. In fact, harsh soaps may actually irritate the anus, especially if you insert a soapy finger to wash out the sensitive anal canal. Any kind of natural glycerin soap (limited ingredients, no perfumes) will do the trick.

If you're engaging in external play only, you won't need to do much else. You don't even need to take a full shower. If you can manage it safely, just hang your butt over the edge of the bathtub and wash that area only (or your genitals too, if you like) for a quick-and-not-so-dirty way to clean your back door. Alternatively, if you'd rather get just your lower half wet, use a detachable showerhead for a cleaning that's less time-consuming than a full shower. If water is inaccessible or inconvenient, try alcohol-free wipes, which are a great backup. They won't get you quite as clean as water will, but they're good in a pinch and are much more effective than toilet paper, which balls up and leaves bits of dirty lint behind.

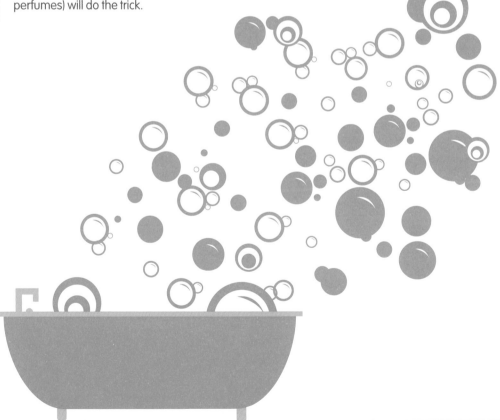

Internally

Some anal adventurers like to get their insides squeaky clean, too—and that's not as difficult (or uncomfortable) as you'd think. A basic enema can help clean out the rectum, which means that anything up to 7 inches (17.7 cm) long that's inserted into the rectum should be free of poop traces. An internal cleaning is best done in the morning or on an empty stomach and after a BM if possible. This makes it a much more comfortable process. For this procedure, you'll need either a rectal/bulb syringe for regular douching, or an enema for a single use. Both are available from the drugstore. The syringe tends to hold more water, which means it's more time-efficient since it requires fewer refills. If you're using a regular enema, know that enema bottles are prefilled, containing laxative ingredients designed to stimulate a BM. If this is not your intent, empty the contents down the sink and rinse out the bottle before you get started.

Fill the syringe or bottle with warm water. Some prefer salt water because it's more like our body composition, and regular water can draw electrolytes from the body. To make a salt solution, combine 1 teaspoon of pure sea salt and 1 liter of water. Run the water until it reaches a comfortable temperature—not too hot, and not too cold. Test the water's temperature on the inside of your arm, just as you'd test milk before giving it to a baby. When in doubt, err on the side of cool rather than hot. You don't want to burn your insides! (Anyway, as long as the water isn't *really* cold, it shouldn't result in much discomfort.)

Fill the syringe or enema bottle with water, and put a little lube at the tip to help it slide inside. Sit on the toilet, squat, or bend over; insert the tip; and then squeeze the water in. If you are using a reusable rectal syringe, be careful not to suck the dirty water back into the empty syringe after expelling the water. Hold the syringe tightly while you withdraw it. Make sure you wash out the insides well when you are done. The advantage of a Fleet enema is that it is disposable; thus there's less concern about cleanliness. You can either let the water out of your butt immediately, or hold it in while you refill the bottle and then your butt a couple more times in order to fill up your rectum more completely. When you are full enough, sit on the toilet and let the water flow out. After a few rinses, you'll know that you're done when all that comes out is clean water. This process can take as little as 5 minutes and can be an effective way to prep for internal anal pleasure.

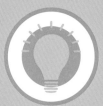

Tap or bottled, sir?

Because the rectum is so absorbent, some regular enema users prefer to use pure distilled water and/or salt water, much in the same way that you might choose to drink purified water only, since most tap water is treated with chemicals like chlorine and fluoride. And because what the rectum absorbs during an enema is not filtered through the digestive tract, some people believe that chemicals are more harmful when they're ingested this way.

FROM OUR SURVEY

" *Commercially-available enemas, like Fleet, are preferred for a quick clean-out. A rectal syringe is also helpful to ensure that the rectum is fully cleaned out prior to play. A deep cleanse is nice, but it's a bit more time-consuming and has to be done several hours before the action to ensure that cleansing and draining is complete.* "

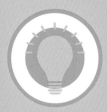

Toxic tushies

This one's pretty high up on the list of Worst Ideas Ever: Don't put alcohol or caffeine up your butt. It'll be absorbed into your bloodstream quickly, but without being filtered by your digestive system—and that means it can be dangerous, and even poisonous. When it comes to caffeinated or alcoholic beverages, be sure to stick to the other end (your mouth, that is!) so that your taste buds get to enjoy the process, too.

For deeper penetration, or for loosening the stools that accumulate further inside in the colon, some folks use an enema bag. If you've never seen one before, it looks like a hot water bottle with a long tube attached. Here's how to use it: Grab your enema bag, lube, and whatever type of water you plan to use, and head to a private bathroom. Decide on a position that's comfortable for you, whether that's lying in the tub on your back, lying on your side, or bent over. (Actually, it's worth pointing out that it's easier to hold in the water if your body is horizontal. When you're standing up, gravity puts more pressure on your sphincters as they work to hold in the contents.) Next, find a hook on which to hang the enema bag. The enema bag should be around 2 or 3 feet (0.5 or 1 m) higher than your butt, so if you're planning to lie on the ground, hanging it from a doorknob can be convenient. Then, follow these steps:

1. Fill the bag with the water (approximately 1 liter) and attach the tube.

2. Hang the bag on the hook (or doorknob) and let the water flow out slowly to eliminate any air bubbles in the tube. Once the water comes out in a steady, slow stream, clamp the tube close to the bag to stop the flow.

3. Get into position, lubricate your anus and the tip of the enema, and insert the tip about 2 inches (5 cm), if possible.

4. Release the clamp slowly to fill your colon gradually. If you fill it too quickly, it can create discomfort and trigger your defecation reflex. If you feel cramping, stop the water flow and breathe deeply. Let out your breath slowly until the discomfort subsides. Massaging your abdomen can help relieve discomfort, too.

5. Fill your colon until you feel full but comfortable, and hold it for a few minutes. Some people can take two quarts of water—but never force yourself to take more than feels right for you.

6. Move around. Stand up if you can, and/or massage your intestines. Massage counterclockwise while the water is filling your colon. Massage clockwise as it exits. This helps to lessen cramping and loosen anything solid so that it can flow out with the water when you release it.

7. Sit on the toilet, let it go, and let it flow!

This process is lengthier than a standard enema and needs to be completed well in advance of sex play. While most of the fluid will evacuate immediately, it can take up to an hour for the full flushing effect to finish up. And you don't want to be in the midst of sex when the final rush happens! Stay close to a bathroom until everything has come out. While you're waiting, wash the enema bag and nozzle and hang them to dry so that mold won't build up inside. Never share your equipment with anyone else; you don't want to swap your individual intestinal bacteria for your partner's. For more detailed information on this process, go online and visit www.enemabag.com.

FROM OUR SURVEY

I opt for an enema with a small shower. Doing it with a partner gives a big sensation of liberty.

Your intestinal tract has its own mucosal and bacterial balance, which means that regular enema use can throw off the rectum's natural ecology and wash away some of the protective mucosa. If vigorous anal play happens soon after a cleaning, there's a greater likelihood of discomfort, tearing, and transmission of infection, because the rectum's natural protective lining is no longer present. That's why it's a good idea to wait a couple of hours post-enema before having sex so your body has a chance to rebuild some of the lining. Some people also eat yogurt with live acidophilus after cleansing to replace the healthy bacteria that get washed away. It's best not to use enemas too often. While there are no official guidelines, once or twice a month should be safe for most folks.

Shower power

If you're an advanced anal sex player, you can also use a diverter attachment to direct water from the shower into your rectum. But it's not quite that easy; there's a danger that the force and speed of the water is significantly higher, and you don't know exactly how much fluid you're using. Wait until you have a lot of experience with enema bags to know how your abdomen feels when it's full of water before you embark on this internal cleansing adventure. And do plenty of research before you give it a go; don't do it until you feel confident that you can try it safely. No matter how great anal sex feels, risking your health for a squeaky-clean back door just isn't worth it!

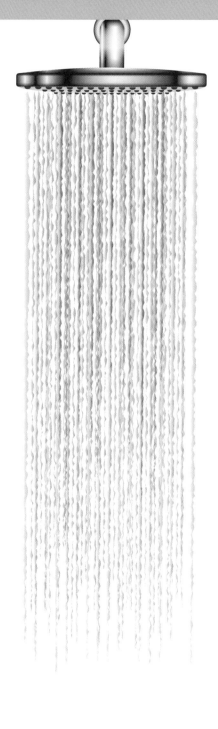

FROM OUR SURVEY

" *I'm not interested in the idea that sex should be sanitized. I want my lover's cum, sweat, tears, blood, shit, and ejaculate. I want my sex to be dirty and raw. I don't want anyone I have sex with—including the sex I have with myself—to feel like their ass is only fuckable or lovable if it's been washed down.* "

FROM OUR SURVEY

"I don't remove any hair from my butt, because I find hair to be super-sexy. Especially furry butt hair."

TO SHAVE OR NOT TO SHAVE?

That truly is the question—for some anal sex aficionados, at least. Some people do like to remove the hair on their faces, armpits, legs, genitals, or butts. Your preference is your own, but there are advantages and disadvantages to each. Remember, though, that the hair on your butt is there for a reason. It prevents foreign particles from entering the body (just like nasal hair does); it reduces friction and chafing; and it keeps the area dry and well-ventilated. I've heard lots of anecdotes from people who were unpleasantly surprised by post-shaving discomfort. Shaving can cause uncomfortable sweat accumulation between the butt cheeks, which in turn can lead to stronger butt smells, noisier farts, and red marks from chafing. That can be pretty disconcerting, especially if you decided to shave to be cleaner and more comfortable! Plus, as hair grows back, red bumps and ingrown hairs can crop up. Use a loofah or exfoliating cloth to help minimize ingrown hairs, and reach for cornstarch or talcum powder to reduce the moisture between shaven cheeks.

Is shaving worth it, then? Why would anyone even *want* to remove butt hair?

There are three main reasons: appearance, sensitivity, and cleanliness. Some folks like to present their partners with a hairless butt because they like the way it looks. Also, hair reduces sensation levels, so when there's no hair in the way, you have easy, direct access to anal skin. Now, this doesn't mean that hairy butts don't feel anything—they sure do! It's just that hair creates an extra layer between the anus and the finger or tongue that's caressing it. Finally, a hairless butt is a usually a cleaner butt. Toilet paper is great for cleaning up after a BM, but it sometimes leaves behind bits of poop, or dingleberries, that attach themselves to anal hair. Without hair, there are no dried dingleberries to contend with. But then again, pre-sex showers can eliminate them, too, so they're certainly not an insurmountable obstacle. And hairless bums have their downsides—so, ultimately, you'll have to come up with your own answer to the "To shave or not to shave?" question. You might also consider trimming your anal hair instead of shaving it off completely; it can maximize the benefits while minimizing the drawbacks of either extreme. Use a beard trimmer or body groomer, which lets you choose how close a trim you want.

How to shave your butt in nine easy steps

1. If your hair is thick and/or long, consider using a beard trimmer or body groomer first to get rid of the bulk of the hair. Otherwise, you'll clog your razor and spend a lot of time rinsing and repeating.

2. Take a hot, soapy shower or bath to soften the hairs.

3. Lie on your back with a mirror between your legs, or squat over a mirror. Since you can't get too close to the area to get a good look, a magnifying mirror is a big help. After shaving your butt a few times, you may be able to just feel around and shave safely sans mirror. But use one until you get the hang of it. (Or ask your partner to do it for you!)

4. Lather up with your shaving gel or cream of choice.

5. One at a time, pull each cheek aside as you shave each one.

6. Shave in the same direction as the hair growth if you have sensitive skin. Shaving against the grain will give you a closer shave.

7. Remove the hair from your razor frequently as you work.

8. Rinse the whole area and dry it off. Some people use aloe vera or antiseptic post-shave treatments to soothe the skin and reduce irritation. Antiseptic also closes the pores and kills bacteria.

9. Use a loofah in the shower for a few days afterward to prevent ingrown hairs. Regular shaving will also prevent the short, prickly hairs from chafing your butt cheeks.

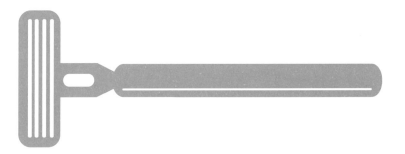

FROM OUR SURVEY

" *A nice, clean surface facilitates rimming. Hair can get pulled and can ruin a play session.* "

You can choose to shave your whole butt, or just your anal area. Lots of different tools can do the trick, so you may have to experiment to see what works best for you, depending on the amount of hair and its coarseness and on your skin's sensitivity.

Many people champion electric razors, which minimize bumps and itching. For wet shaving, folks have different preferences. Some use shaving gel, moisturizing shaving cream, or cocoa-butter lotion. And some recommend using a fresh razor blade every time, while others suggest sticking with one that's been used once or twice. (But whatever you do, don't press down on the razor as you shave, or you'll take off the top layer of skin.) Rinse regularly, and don't pass over the same area too many times. Consider asking your partner to shave you; it can be both erotic and practical since your partner can see what she or he is doing much more easily than you can!

If you are having sex with someone who may have a sexually transmitted infection (STI), you might want to wait a day or two before engaging in anal play to give any cuts or nicks time to heal, since cuts like these are an easy avenue for STI transmission.

Do you want smooth, hairless skin without the hassle of shaving? Here are some other ways to remove butt hair.

Waxing

This is hard to do for yourself. You can ask a friend or partner to help if you get the right equipment, but lots of waxing fans think it's better to see a professional—he or she will have had plenty of experience (not to mention better equipment). Waxers also love the fact that their hair usually grows back more slowly than it would after shaving—and the new hair usually feels softer, too. The downside, of course, is that it's more painful and more expensive. As with shaving, it's best to wax 24–48 hours prior to sex to allow the small bumps and sores to heal.

Electrolysis

Allegedly more permanent than shaving or waxing, electrolysis is also quite painful and expensive and can be performed only by a trained professional. The advantage, though, is that the process kills the hair follicles, which means that less hair grows back each time— thus each subsequent visit is cheaper, and you don't need to go as often once you have it done a few times.

Laser hair removal

This is also a more permanent option than shaving or waxing—but laser hair removal is the most expensive choice when it comes to de-furring. Like electrolysis, it needs to be done by a professional and is painful, but it's a much faster process since the hairs are treated collectively, not individually. Try another option at least once before you go for laser hair removal since it's a pretty permanent choice. Hair is less likely to grow back afterward.

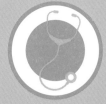

Stay away from depilatories

Never use chemical depilatories near your anus. Depilatories are convenient, easy, and time-efficient, but their ingredients can harm sensitive anal tissue. Besides, they're not very effective for removing coarser, thicker hair.

CONCERNS ABOUT BLEACHING

I'm hesitant to write about the process of bleaching anal skin in case it seems like I'm endorsing the practice. My philosophy is that it's best to celebrate and enjoy our bodies as they are, without altering them to make them conform to some unrealistic, uniform version of "beauty." But the reality is that some folks do bleach their anal skin (as well as the skin on other parts of their bodies). The results, however, are mixed and may be dangerous. If you're considering bleaching any part of your body, do plenty of research first so that you can make a fully informed choice.

It's also important to understand that the skin on your genitals and butt may be a different color than other parts of your body, and that's perfectly normal. These natural variations in skin color are what make us beautiful and unique. And while it might be reasonable for a partner to make requests about cleanliness and hygiene before engaging in anal play, asking someone else to perform permanent—and possibly dangerous—body modifications like bleaching is insensitive, unfair, and unreasonable.

Admire yourself with a mirror

Why not find out what you look like "down there"? Squat over a mirror or lie on your back with a mirror between your legs, and then revel in the beauty of your rosebud. Feel around while you're looking in the mirror, as well, so that you can observe your body's responses to touch. Having a good sense of what your butt looks like can help you feel less vulnerable when you're showing it to a partner, too. It'll be easier to relax into the pleasure when you're confident that everything is clean and ready to go.

FROM OUR SURVEY

" *I've never bleached my butt, and I won't. I accept the colors of my body, and I don't want to be with someone who insists I change what I am to have sex with me.* "

SEXUALLY TRANSMITTED INFECTIONS (STIS) AND SAFER SEX

Even if you're in a monogamous relationship, you need to be mindful of infections that can be transmitted during anal play and of how to have safer sex. Remember that if you already have one STI, the resulting sores make you more likely to contract another. So always play it safe!

A good rule of thumb is to use condoms or gloves on anything that goes inside a butt (and that goes for penises/outies, toys, fingers, and hands). If you have a cut, wait up to 2 days for it to heal before exposing it to anal play; this will prevent infections from entering your bloodstream. If you aren't sure whether a sore on your hand, butt, or genitals is healed or not, squeeze a little lemon juice or alcohol onto it for an instant reading. Even a small sting tells you that your wound is still open.

Use dental dams to cover the external anal area during oral-anal pleasure. A dam can prevent you from ingesting fecal matter. It can also protect your partner if you subsequently move to the vagina and vulva, potentially spreading parasites, bacteria, or STIs.

Even if you're already sharing sexual fluids with your partner and aren't concerned about transmitting STIs, you still need to take precautions when it comes to anal sex. Don't share anal toys with a partner, because each person's intestinal bacteria are slightly different and may be upset by the introduction of foreign bacteria. And oral-anal play is a concern for everyone, since we all carry E. coli in our BMs.

If you're not using a condom during anal intercourse, bits of poop may become trapped in the urethra of a penis/outie and can cause urethritis, which is more unpleasant and annoying than it is dangerous, but definitely something you'll want to avoid. If you have a penis, to help rid the urethra of bacteria, always urinate after anal sex if you don't ejaculate during it. And take care if you wash your penis after anal sex with the intention of putting it inside a vagina or mouth. Bacteria can stick in the opening to your urethra and can still infect your partner if you didn't pee or ejaculate to wash them away.

Lubricant makes sex more pleasurable, but it's also very helpful in preventing STI transmission because it reduces friction, which helps prevent sensitive tissues from tearing. Everyone has a favorite lubricant, but because of the absorptive qualities of the rectum, stay away from lubes that contain chemicals or scents your body could absorb. Most people prefer a thick lubricant for anal play due to its staying power. Get one that comes in a pump, which makes relubing so much easier. Some people even put a condom over their lube bottles so that any juices and STIs that linger on the bottle are easily done away with when the condom is removed during cleanup.

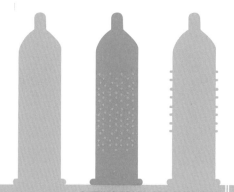

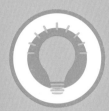

HIV and circumcision

The foreskin on a penis keeps the penis's head, or glans, moist and more sensitive to touch. Conflicting studies disagree on whether uncircumcised men are more at risk for contracting HIV than their circumcised counterparts. In any case, all people with penises, circumcised or not, can greatly reduce the risk to themselves and their partners by using condoms during anal sex. If you're not using condoms, washing the penis after sex decreases the risk slightly by reducing the amount of time that the virus is present on the head of the penis.

FROM OUR SURVEY

" *"I have had the pleasure of intestinal parasites, which you don't usually think about when you think of STIs. It's more of an infestation than infection . . . Not so uncommon if you share a bed with pets or kids. They're treated with meds, but you have to work through some psychology to get back in the game.* "

Steering Clear of STIs and Other Health Risks

Like any type of sex, anal sex does carry some health risks. Practicing safer sex can help you avoid the following:

E. coli, shigella, and parasites can be transmitted from poop to your mouth. To prevent transmission, wash the anal area well before oral-anal play and/or use a dental dam. Wash penises and toys thoroughly after anal play and before putting them into mouths or vaginas.

Hepatitis A and B are also transmitted through feces. Wash the anal area well before oral-anal play and/or use a dental dam as a barrier. Again, always wash penises and toys thoroughly after anal play and before putting them into mouths. (Vaccinations for hepatitis A and B are available, and vaccination is especially recommended if you're traveling to a part of world with poor sanitation, so it's good protection for both purposes.)

HIV is transmitted through blood, vaginal secretions, semen, and rectal mucosal lining, as well as breast milk. Using condoms and gloves for any internal play, and dams for any external play where blood is present, is critical to preventing HIV transmission. If a condom breaks, or if you think you may have been exposed to HIV in any other way, taking post-exposure prophylaxis, or PEP, within 72 hours may help prevent infection.

Chlamydia, gonorrhea, and syphilis can be contracted through anal intercourse and can lead to complications such as pelvic inflammatory disease or PID, infertility, stroke, or meningitis if left untreated with antibiotics. Becoming infected with even one of these places you at a higher risk of contracting other STIs. Use condoms to prevent transmission.

"I have baby wipes around in case I want to clean up without going to the bathroom. Baby wipes soak up fluids and have some cleaning effects, too. Their moistness makes for easier cleaning up of sticky sex fluids as well. I also keep tissues around to hold used toys."

Herpes is transmitted by skin-to-skin contact, and the resulting lesions may develop in or around the anus. Once acquired, it lives in the same place in your body and causes regular or no outbreaks, and it's contagious during and just before an outbreak. About 50 to 80 percent of adults in the United States have herpes, but as many as 90 percent of people who are infected don't know that they have it. Prevent the spread of herpes by using condoms or gloves for internal play, and gloves and dental dams for external play. Take care not to place a gloved hand anywhere else on the body after internal or external play.

Human papillomavirus (HPV, or warts) can be contracted by touching the warts, which develop on the penis and in the rectum as well as in the vagina and on the cervix. HPV can linger on sex toys for over 24 hours, even after they have been washed. There are over one hundred strains of HPV, and some of them can lead to cancer. Luckily, there are vaccines for up to four of the most common—and cancer-inducing—strains. Most sexually active people are likely to contract at least one strain of HPV by the age of thirty, but most strains of HPV are fought off by the body in the same way your immune system fights off a cold or flu. Prevent HPV by using condoms and gloves for internal play and dental dams for external play. Women should get regular Pap smear tests, which screen for HPV, among other things. Those who engage in anal sex with new partners can also get an anal Pap smear to help detect HPV.

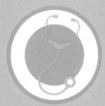

High-risk pleasure

The prevalence of HIV in rectal mucosa is quite high—even higher than in blood or semen. That means it's possible to transmit HIV via anal intercourse, even if no tearing takes place. Both partners—the penetrator and the penetratee—can transmit it to one other, so get tested regularly, and always use condoms.

SAFER SEX IS BETTER SEX

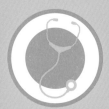 As with crossing the street, so with sex: safety first! Actually, there is no such thing as "safe" sex, since the only way to be completely safe is to abstain from any kind of sexual activity. Period. But that's not much fun, and lots of people have safer sex that is totally hot and extremely satisfying. And those of us with STIs can still have fabulous sexual lives while keeping ourselves and our partners as safe as possible. However, it's important to know and consider the risks and to understand how to play as safely as you can while having fun with a partner. When in doubt, check with your local sexual health clinic or reliable online resources.

Here are some basic guidelines.

Get yourself tested regularly.
If you're not comfortable discussing this issue with your family doctor, visit an anonymous sexual health clinic. Those clinics will be able to provide you with the latest information on protecting yourself, depending on your sexual activities, your health, and your partner or partners' health. If you have a regular partner, go together. That way, you'll both have the same (accurate!) information. Make it a date!

Use condoms, gloves, and dental dams.
I can't say it often enough! Always use condoms on penises/outies and toys that you plan to insert in a vagina/innie, anus, or mouth. Use gloves on your hands, especially if you have cuts on them. Use dental dams for oral sex on a vulva and/or anus. If you are allergic or sensitive to latex, there are non-latex options; just remember that lambskin condoms protect against pregnancy but not STIs like HIV, so use polyurethane or polyisoprene non-latex options instead.

Use lube.
Lubricant makes everything glide more smoothly. It feels good, but more importantly, it prevents tearing in the sensitive rectal or vaginal lining (and prevents tears in condoms, dams, and gloves, too). Lube also minimizes pain from friction caused by sores that might already be in and on your body. Condoms—even lubricated ones—and gloves need extra lube. Any way you slice it, with only small amounts of mucosa in the rectum, lube is essential to pleasurable anal play.

Don't use nonoxynol-9.
Nonoxynol-9 is a spermicidal compound found in some lubricants, condoms, and other contraceptive products. While it helps prevent pregnancy and kill HIV, its intense cleaning power irritates your sensitive tissues, reducing pleasure and making it easier for any infection to pass into your body through the small sores it often creates. The negative effects of the irritation outweigh any nonoxynol-9's benefits. Use spermicide only when preventing pregnancy and when you are not concerned about STI transmission. Another alternative is to put some inside of a glove or condom so that you don't experience the downsides of rectum irritation, but if the condom or glove breaks, you gain the benefits of its HIV-fighting qualities.

Talk about it.
Have a frank discussion about safe sex with each new partner. Come up with a speech about your sexual health, boundaries, and safer sex practices and rehearse it ahead of time—with a willing friend, if you like. Getting in the habit of talking about safer sex will make you feel confident about bringing it up with a partner. And the more confident you are, the more likely you are to articulate your safer-sex boundaries and practices—and to stick to them.

POST-SEX CLEAN-UP

FROM OUR SURVEY

" *I'm obsessed with clean. I love gloves because they're sexy (nothing is hotter to me than putting lubed, gloved fingers in someone's bum!).* "

After sex, all you want to do is chill out and enjoy the afterglow as your brain and body are flooded with endorphins. And that means post-sex cleanup can be a bit of a drag. But a few easy preventative measures can minimize the amount of time and effort you invest in après-sex tidying. A cover for the bed (or wherever you like to have sex) is almost essential. Disposable chucks or blue pads from the medical supply store are handy; they absorb fluids, which makes them a fast, cheap way to clean up in one fell swoop. A more environmentally friendly option would be a washable, reusable towel or blanket. If you ask me, the sexiest eco-option is the washable, waterproof Liberator Throe (www. liberator.com), which can be tossed straight into the wash after sex. It's also handy to have towels and/or baby wipes around. They're great for cleaning individual body parts mid- and post-sex, when you're not ready to get up and take a shower. If you want to postpone a major cleanup until later, that's fine. Just wrap all the toys and towels in your choice of bedcover or put them in your Sex Pot (a pot that can be used later for boiling sterilizable toys), and leave them on the floor until you're ready to deal with them.

Prepping for anal sex is completely your call. Some folks do almost nothing at all to get ready, while others find that extensive prep is a super-pleasurable part of the process. Be aware of safer-sex considerations. Apart from that, the details are up to you. But I'll leave you with one caveat: if you're planning a date that might involve partnered anal pleasure, try the typical romantic-dinner-followed-by-sex option—just do it in reverse. Even a little food and drink can trigger elimination, so you may prefer to have sex first and eat afterward. (It can even be more fun that way; you'll have the opportunity to work up an appetite, then enjoy great post-sex conversation over a romantic meal or snacks in bed!) Now that you're ready for anal play, chapter 4 will show you how to get started.

Chapter 4

THE APPROACH:
EXTERNAL ANAL PLAY

Anal sex: Isn't it all about putting *that* in *there*? Not necessarily. Let's step outside of the proverbial box for a bit. When we envision anal sex, we usually form a mental image of a penis inside a butt—which is, of course, an extremely limiting model. As with any other type of sex, the possibilities for pleasure are endless, and they're not dependent on penetration, either. My first anal pleasure teacher, Chester, used to teach at the Body Electric School, where he'd hold weeklong anal play workshops—and he'd spend the first 2 (or more!) days focusing on external pleasure only. "Traditional" sex can be a little too goal-oriented when the emphasis is on getting or "winning" access to certain parts of the body, or on penetration, ejaculation, and orgasm (in that order). But sex is so much more interesting and fulfilling when it's about a journey rather than a destination. Most of the time, slower is better; even simply holding still to notice and feel the subtleties of the moment during sex play can be surprisingly profound.

So we're going to start out slowly. Whether you've tried anal play already or not, a great place to start experimenting is in the bathtub or shower.

While you're doing your daily scrub-a-dub routine, lather up and take an extra minute or two to feel the outside of your rosebud with a finger. Try making circles with your finger; move it up and down or side to side. Place a little pressure on the opening, and breathe into the sensations. (Our instincts tell us to hold our breath when we try something new or scary or when we're feeling insecure—but just breathing deeply can be a surprisingly effective way to relax and be mindful of the new sensations you're experiencing.)

When you're ready to focus on anal play specifically, grab some lube and toys and make yourself comfortable. You may find that exploring on your own is the easiest way to start. While playing with a partner is fabulous, knowing what you like beforehand and being able to communicate that to your partner generally makes any sexual experience better. Solo play may feel less awkward and self-conscious than partnered play—at least at first.

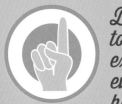

Do I have to start with external play every time I have anal sex?

Nope. Many anal enthusiasts enjoy intercourse or other internal play quite easily without all of the warm-up. But most of them have had to work their way up to it. Pain-free anal sessions teach your anus to trust that whatever's entering it will feel great. Thus, it easily opens and welcomes the incoming toy, finger, or penis as well as the accompanying pleasure. If you take your time and use external pleasure to give your anus a warm-up, it'll eventually relax, making internal play painless. Once the anus trusts you, you can often enjoy a penis or similarly sized toy right off the bat with only pleasure as your guide. But external stimulation still feels great on its own, so why skip it just because you can? Besides, it's also a great technique for teasing your partner until she or he begs you for more!

FROM OUR SURVEY

❝ *"Talk for a while before you even undress. And laugh! Make jokes, tell fantasies, share concerns. Don't rush. Poke around with fingers very gently. Massage, massage, massage. Warm up to each other. And discover each other's bodies like you have all the time in the world to learn.* ❞

Why bother with external anal play before taking the plunge inside? Here are two great reasons:

1. It feels great. External play is part of the anal experience, and it's so worth it. In fact, it's so pleasurable that for some folks, anal sex is about external play only. You might decide that external pleasure is a step on the journey—or you might decide that it's also your final destination. It's up to you!

2. It helps make internal play more pleasurable—or even possible. You may have already experienced this common scenario: Your partner tried to put a finger, toy, or penis inside, but it either wouldn't go in or felt painful when it did. Well, there's a good reason for that. In the moment, your mind wanted to trust your partner, your heart wanted to trust your partner, but your anus was not ready to trust your partner. Your anus has a mind of its own and won't relax on command, especially if you've had painful anal sex before or if you're afraid that sex might be painful this time. Some people call this anticipatory pain. Technical terms aside, though, this experience is all too common. In fact, many regular anal players tell me that they expect that anal penetration will be painful, and then they suffer through it—sometimes throughout the entire encounter. And that's a shame, because this type of pain can easily be avoided. This is where external play comes in. For lots of folks, it's the key to pleasurable internal play. Personally, if I'm with a partner, I like to spend at least 10 minutes on external pleasure (and even longer if I'm with a partner who's really nervous or who's had previous painful or unsuccessful experiences). This attention to pleasure helps the anus relax and trust, and it makes it hungry for more. After some external play, a finger or finger-width toy can usually slide into the butt easily and comfortably.

RELAX BEFORE YOU HEAD FOR THE BACK DOOR

You'll have a much better anal experience if you relax before you approach your butt. If you're short on time, or if you simply want to get right to it, go for it—but don't be surprised if it takes a little longer for your body to sync into the pleasure. Why not take a bath, meditate, give yourself (or each other) an orgasm, or start with a full-body massage? When you're ready, bring your awareness to your rear end by squeezing your anal sphincter muscles (as though you were holding in a bowel movement), then relaxing them. Inhale deeply a few times, and imagine that you're breathing in through your anus; feel your breath travel up your spine, and watch it flow out through your mouth.

Butt massage is a great way to move toward the anal area. Here are some techniques to get you started. (Some of these moves are easier if your partner is willing to give you a hand!)

Vibrating hands

Place the fingertips of each hand somewhere on the semicircle that extends from your tailbone, around the sides and along the crease of the butt, back toward the crack. Push in with the tips of your three middle fingers and vibrate them to make the butt jiggle. (If you're doing this for your partner, reassure her or him that everybody's butt jiggles, no matter how big or small it is!) Continue to vibrate your fingers in the same spot for 10–15 seconds, then shift to another spot along the semicircle of the butt, and vibrate your fingers again.

Big Cs

You'll want to use some massage oil for this classic Swedish massage technique! Form a C shape with each hand, thumbs down, while putting pressure on the butt with the thumb, pinkie, and heel of your hand. Move one hand toward the other, and then glide it back in the other direction while your other hand moves forward. Focus on one butt cheek at a time. Pretend that each cheek is a clock, and move each hand from the outer numbers in toward the middle and back again, ending on a different number with each rotation.

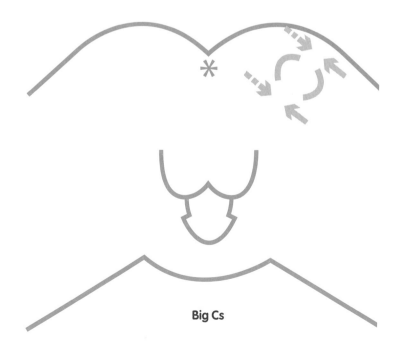

Big Cs

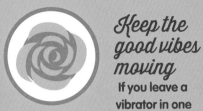

Keep the good vibes moving

If you leave a vibrator in one spot—on your anus or anywhere else—for longer than 15 seconds, your nerve endings will become acclimatized to the sensations and will start to tune them out. To counter this, move your vibrator from time to time. Even just a slight movement will stimulate new nerves, keeping them tingly and excited.

FROM OUR SURVEY

" My first internal anal play experience was with a British dominatrix. She was licking my asshole with her tongue and playing with my anus with her finger while I lay on my back. She was very enthusiastic about it, and it was much more sensitive than I expected. "

ANAL-FOCUSED PLAY

After you've indulged in a little massage, you might feel ready to move closer to the anus. Now it's time to relax your rosebud using vibration, tongues, hands, and fingers.

Vibration

Already got a vibrating toy or two? Dig them out of the drawer, because they're the perfect place to start. Note that the following techniques are purely external, so there's no need to use a "butt-specific" toy here. Put a condom on the toy (if you'll be using it beyond your butt), lube it up, and start on low speed. Sensations on the rosebud feel really intense, so don't ramp up the speed too soon. Move the toy around in circles, up and down, and from side to side; alternatively, use it to tap your rosebud gently, roll it back and forth, and try placing a little pressure on your anus. Experiment and see what feels great.

If you're exploring with a partner, avoid placing the toy against the anal opening in such a way that you could easily or accidentally push it in. You want the rosebud to relax as much as possible. Even though *you* know you're not going to push it in, your partner's rosebud doesn't. And if the well-lubed toy is poking at the anal opening, your partner might be thinking, *I'll bet it will slip in. I know we said we'd stick to external play only—but I just know it's going to slip in!* Thoughts like these will make your partner tense and anxious. So, unless your partner craves penetration and you're just trying to tease her or him, be sure to place a toy flat against the rosebud so that it's lying in the crack of the butt. This way, your partner can easily relax into the lovely sensations.

" *Our physical chemistry was already hot, but she when offered to have anal sex with me for the first time, we both got extremely excited! It began with her lying down on her stomach on my bed, and me slowly eating her pussy out from behind. I licked up, down, and all around, lubricating her pussy and anus with my tongue, and relaxing her ass muscles. Then she asked me to play with her anus with my finger—which I did, after I added a thick dollop of lubrication to my pinkie. Slowly, I tickle-rimmed her to relax her more, and enjoyed learning the contours and reactions of her fleshy backside, healthy thighs, and curvy hips. After playing with her pussy and anus for about 15 minutes, I slid my penis between her bum cheeks and got cozy up against her body. I started getting an erection—and an inkling of what all the anal hoopla is all about.* "

Tongue and mouth

It's actually hard to do anything with your mouth that *isn't* pleasurable, since it's naturally wet, soft, and flexible. And, unlike toys and fingers, using your tongue can often make it easier for the receiver to relax, because even if a toy or finger slips in, it's unlikely to cause pain or penetrate deeply. Tongues are a great place to start when it comes to partnered anal pleasure. (Unfortunately, most of us can't offer oral pleasure to ourselves!)

A few notes on safer oral-anal sex: before you start, if you're not sure when your partner last had a BM, ask her or him. (Or just play in or after the shower following a thorough lathering!) You can also use a dental dam for extra protection against STIs, E. coli, and parasites—or just because you or your partner prefer it. A dental dam is a thin, square piece of latex that offers safer sex plus plenty of pleasure—and other perks! Because we can't see our own butts without getting friendly with a mirror, if we're on the receiving end of external anal play, we may feel shy when our partners get up close and personal with our backsides. If that sounds familiar, a dental dam can help you relax, safe in the knowledge that your partner isn't going to come into contact with any fecal matter. Plus, as you know from chapter 3, dental dams are important if you're playing with a new or casual partner; hepatitis and herpes are easily transmitted through oral-anal stimulation.

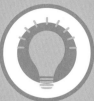

Dental dams and great sex

Lots of folks find that using safer-sex supplies, like condoms and dental dams, diminishes the pleasure of sex. While it's true that barriers do affect sensation levels, there are plenty of ways to maximize the fun. First of all, use a dental dam that's designed for oral sex, not the kind dentists use. Second, be sure to apply some lube to the underside of the dam—the side that'll be pressed against the skin. Third, don't stretch the dam taut over the genital or anal area. Instead, tuck it into all the nooks and crannies, so that all the folds of skin can be stimulated and explored. If you stretch the dam, only the parts that stick out the most will be able to feel the sensations. To get a better picture of this, imagine that you're putting plastic wrap over a cup. If you pull the plastic tight, like a drum, you'll only be able to feel the rim of the cup, not its bottom or sides. But if you relax the plastic wrap and line the bottom and sides of the cup with it, your finger will have access to all of the surfaces. Even though your anus doesn't have crevices that are quite so deep, the same principle applies. So relax the dam, and tuck it into the folds so that all the nerve endings get to partake in the pleasure.

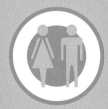

One trans man's effects of testosterone on butt play

During the first few months of transition, I became more and more focused on butt play. Most of my play and fantasies had anal stimulation as a central theme. I found that when my perineal sponge was stimulated by penetration, my cock would get instantly hard. I also found that anal stimulation like rimming and light touch on the anus gave me a great amount of pleasure. I do believe that testosterone has contributed to my changing sexual desires and the increased pleasure I experience during anal play.

—From Carey Gray, owner of Aslan Leather

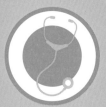

Dangerous drips

If you're lying on your belly, lube or other liquids can drip down from your anus to your vagina—if you have one—bringing harmful bacteria with them. Roll up a towel and place it against your perineum to catch and absorb any errant fluids. This is also a good way to keep hands, fingers, or toys that have been inside the anus from touching the vagina by accident.

FROM OUR SURVEY

I love licking my partner's ass. It's so sensual and intimate. She won't let me go inside of her, but she adores it when my tongue travels from her vagina to her butthole.

Try these techniques with your tongue and lips:

Make circles. They can either be the same size, or you can spiral from small to large and back again.

Suck the anus and the area around it.

Lick the crack of the butt. The length can be long or short; long licks can start at the clitoris or head of the penis and end all the way back at the tailbone.

Flick your tongue, either softly or firmly, over the rosebud.

Pucker your lips, and then stick them out and make a buzzing sound (like the one you made when you were playing with toy cars as a kid).

Vibrate your tongue with your lips slightly parted, as if you were imitating the purring of a cat.

Lick the skin, and then blow on it, as though you were blowing out a candle. The sensation will feel cool.

Lick and then blow from the back of your mouth, as if you were warming up cold hands. The sensation will feel warm.

Place your mouth over your partner's anus, and make any kind of sound. The vibration of your mouth will send ripples of sensation to the area.

Tease your partner. Run your tongue up and down the crack of the butt—but don't let your tongue touch the anus itself.

Add flavored lube, melted chocolate, or your favorite liqueur to the mix. Spread it on, and then lick it off. Just be careful not to allow these edibles near a vagina or urethra since the glycerin or sugar can lead to infections.

FROM OUR SURVEY

As a heterosexual man, anal has been unofficially declared 'the forbidden zone'—that is, until I stopped being ignorant and afraid of exploring, understanding, and appreciating the entirety of my own damn body! I enjoy exploring the delicacy of the ass, and the safety as well as the danger of playing with it. Having my ass licked this year was one of the most exhilarating and delightful sexual experiences I've had in my life, and those adventurous women who have been willing to share that experience with me have taken a special place in my heart and soul.

Use your hands

Hands are so versatile. They can do just about anything. Joseph Kramer's anal massage DVDs (www.eroticmassage.com) are the best resources for learning how to pleasure the butt with your hands. If you want to be a true butt master, getting a copy is one of the best things you can do for yourself (and your partner). Here are some of my favorite moves. (Remember to add lube or massage oil to prevent friction and enhance sensation.)

Stretch It Out. Using two hands, gently pull the skin just to the side of the rosebud in opposite directions. The area is so sensitive that this motion will indirectly stimulate the rosebud's nerve endings.

Variations: Stretch the skin from side to side, from top to bottom, and diagonally. Move your hands super-slowly, and then move them faster and faster. Wiggle your fingers as you pull.

Hands Down. You can use one or both hands for this move. Turn your hand so it's pinkie-down, as if you were about to give someone a handshake. Then lay your hand along the crack of the butt against the rosebud, and glide it down the crack from top to bottom.

Variations: The back of the hand can remain flat, or bend your wrist as you would doing a handshake so that the tips of your fingers, from your pinkie to your index finger, each glide against the rosebud one at a time. You can vibrate your hand as it glides or while holding it in place. You can also hold a vibrator between your thumb and index finger to enhance your vibrations.

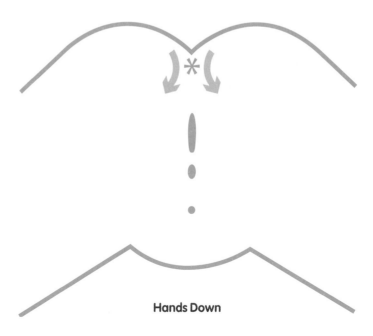

Hands Down

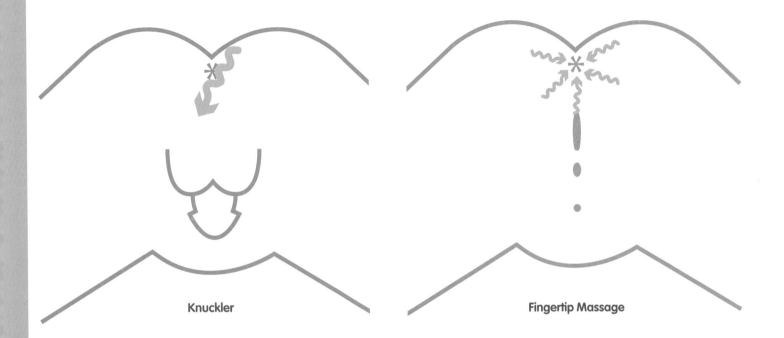

Knuckler

Fingertip Massage

Knuckler. Curl the fingers of one hand gently, and press the backs of your curled fingers against the rosebud. Move your fingers together, or wiggle each finger rhythmically.

Variations: Move your hand up and down along the crack of the butt, or simply leave it in place. Use two hands side by side, or one on top of the other. To vibrate, shake your hand or hold a vibrator in your palm.

Fingertip Massage. Place the backs of your hands against each other, palms out. Wiggle your fingertips against the rosebud.

Variations: Move your hands up and down the crack of the butt, or stay in one place. Place one hand above the other.

FROM OUR SURVEY

" *I convinced my guy to let me use the techniques on the [Joseph Kramer anal massage] DVD. OMG: I have never heard him moan like that. He actually said he might want me to put my finger in next time.* "

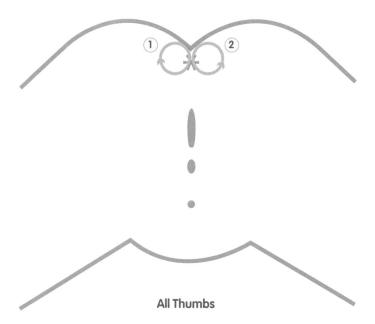

All Thumbs

All Thumbs. Place your left thumb against the rosebud and your right thumb on top of the left one. Rotate your thumbs until the right one is under the left, as if you were twiddling your thumbs. Repeat again and again.

Variations: Make one small circle to the left of the rosebud with the left thumb, followed by a small circle to the right with the right thumb. Do this in such a way that each thumb passes along the rosebud, then circles to the side in opposite directions. Move your thumbs in time to a rhythm, with the left one to the left and the right one to the right of the rosebud.

After you try a few of these techniques, it won't take long for your anus to relax and surrender to pleasure. Go ahead and devote a full session to external play. There's no pressure to do anything except breathe and enjoy. And the more often you engage in anal play, the quicker your body will become used to it, and it'll trust you more easily when you want to approach the anal area again. Pay attention to the thousands of nerve endings at your fingertips—and when you're ready for internal play, you'll find plenty of pleasure there, too. Chapter 5 will show you how.

TAKING THE PLUNGE:
INTERNAL ANAL PLEASURE

We're finally here! Now that you've experimented with external anal pleasure, you're ready to take the next step: internal play. If you're a beginner, you're probably eager to find out what all the fuss is about—is it really *that* good?—and if you're a seasoned anal aficionado, you might be interested in new ways to enjoy penetrative play.

If you've already engaged in many anal play sessions, your body might be well used to the sensations and may easily open up without a lot of foreplay to the pleasure that's knocking at your back door. But you might still want to try a little external seduction first, just because it feels so good. If you're a newbie to anal (or if you've tried it before and didn't like it), you should definitely start with external play first. Revisit the strategies you learned in chapter 4 so that your anus is relaxed, trusting, and hungry before you progress to penetrative pleasure.

When you're ready, this chapter will walk you through each step of internal butt play. You'll see that penetration can—and should—be pain-free. You'll learn how to use butt plugs, and you'll find out why they're an anal player's best friend. I'll also help you embrace the new and sometimes unfamiliar sensations you'll experience—and I'll show you why staying in the present moment and communicating with your partner throughout the experience are the keys to delicious internal pleasure. Finally, you'll get a crash course on how prostate play (for those of us with prostates) can be an awesome addition to your anal sex life.

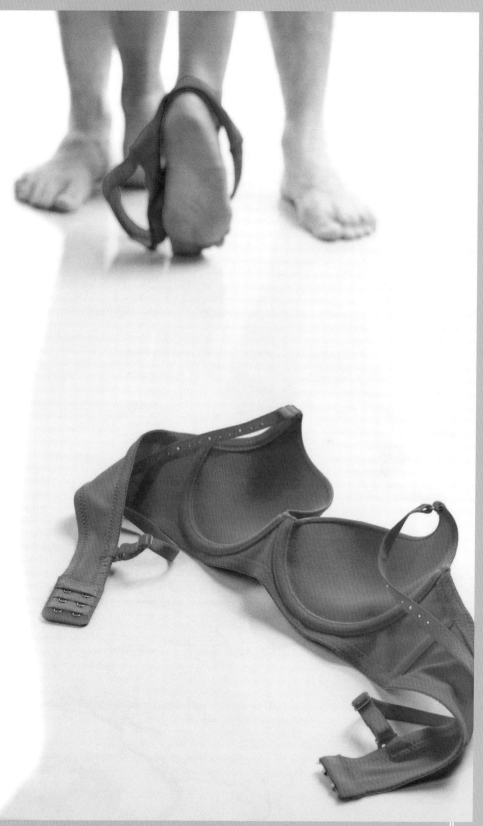

FROM OUR SURVEY

"I'd describe prostate orgasms as feeling very openhearted and involving the whole body. They make me feel hot. They feel like they arise from the core of my being, and not just the tip of my penis. If I have unlimited time for solo play, I might have two to four non-ejaculatory orgasms before I'm so hot and turned on that I want the full screaming release."

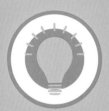

Numb is dumb

Stay away from desensitizing creams or lubes, which are designed to reduce sensation levels. After all, what's the point of having sex if you can't feel it? It's true that you won't feel any pain—but then again, you won't feel any pleasure, either. (What's more, these creams can irritate a condomless penis—or, at best, numb it.) Desensitizing products are actually dangerous, because they prevent you from noticing any harmful tearing or poking. And they may minimize pain *during* sex—but, oh boy, will you ever notice the irritation when the cream's effects have worn off! Instead, go slowly and enjoy every minute of the experience. If you feel pain, stop what you're doing or switch techniques.

INTERNAL PLEASURE: THE BASICS

Before you even think about putting anything into your butt, memorize these four basic rules for safe, pleasurable penetrative play:

Lube, lube, and more lube

It's actually pretty difficult to use too much lube! Most folks prefer to use a thick lube for anal play because it's better at staying in place, which means you don't need to reapply it every 2 minutes. Some anal-play connoisseurs have fancy lube "recipes"—two parts of this lube to one part of that one—and they experiment constantly to find the consistency that works best for them. That's because butts are unique and individual: each one has its own preferences. Some people use a lube shooter (drawn on the next page) to get lube inside the rectum for maximum slipperiness before a toy is inserted. (For more advice on choosing the best lube for you, check out chapter 8.)

Start small

Don't begin your adventure by inserting a penis or large toy, unless of course you are experienced at taking one without pain. A finger, or a toy of similar width, is the perfect place to start. This is so important, because a smooth, enjoyable kickoff to internal anal play ensures that you're relaxed and fully aware of the pleasure. Beginning with a large toy or penis can be overwhelming and can distract you from the good sensations. Think of it like this: If you get a fast, deep massage that moves across your body too quickly, it'll be hard to really sink into feeling the masseur's hands. But a slow massage that focuses on one area of the body at a time lets the brain catch up with the body—hence the profoundly satisfying, deeply felt levels of sensation and pleasure.

FROM OUR SURVEY

We have used numbing products when new to anal play. We no longer do, as she has grown more accustomed to play and no longer has any pain associated with it.

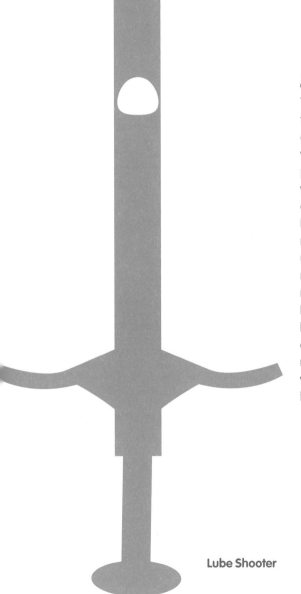

Lube Shooter

Trim your nails

The lining of the rectum and anus is quite fragile and easy to puncture. Some seasoned anal players have a designated finger (DF) with a shorter nail that they use for safe penetration. This is especially handy when a vulva is close by because there's less chance of the wrong finger going in next door. In the heat of the moment, it can be tough to remember which finger you put where, so using a DF leads to fewer mistakes. Gloves make everything smoother, but long, sharp nails can even puncture through a glove. Here's what to do if you want to keep your long nails: tear a cotton ball in half, and insert one half under and around the tip of the nail—then put a glove on over your hand. This will protect the anus and rectum, but you'll still be able to feel your way around.

Pay attention to pain

So many folks—even those who engage in regular anal play—resign themselves to the expectation that anal sex will hurt. But that simply isn't true. Slow down your expectations and your movements, and allow the pleasure to simply happen. If you force yourself (and your anus) to endure pain, your anus will remember: it stores these memories for self-preservation later, and you'll be less likely to relax into anal play the next time you try. The anticipatory pain locked into your sphincters' memory will actually keep your butt from opening. So if something hurts, adjust your movements until things feel good again.

Listen to your butt. If you experience pain, change your actions immediately. Stop any movement of fingers or toys, breathe deeply, and add lube. When the pain subsides, adjust your technique by altering the angle, depth, size, and/or speed of penetration. If you still feel pain, withdraw the toy or finger slowly and focus on external play—or switch to other erogenous zones and leave the anal play for another time. There are always other opportunities. Besides, if you show your anus that you listen to its needs, it'll be more likely to trust you the next time, secure in the knowledge that pleasure is the goal and that any unintended pain will be short-lived.

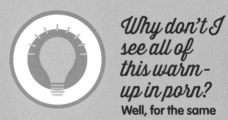

Why don't I see all of this warm-up in porn?

Well, for the same reasons that you don't see every moment of a character's life in a regular Hollywood movie. In the same way that mainstream filmmakers omit seconds, minutes, or even years from a character's storyline, most porn films skip over the "unnecessary" parts. Porn is designed to turn on the viewer, and most directors don't think viewers will be aroused by a slow, gradual buildup. Plus, they edit out the parts where the performers get "fluffed" or aroused off-camera—or, less sexy, the parts where they fart or add more lube. Ultimately, porn isn't an accurate play-by-play of how most folks enjoy sex—anal or otherwise!

FROM OUR SURVEY

" *Anal sex can potentially be painful, but for the most part, if you do it right, it shouldn't be. Pay attention to your body and decide for yourself where that line is, and follow that. Communicate what is painful and what your needs are. A good partner will listen.* **"**

PAIN-FREE PENETRATION

Going pain-free is generally the goal. Most people are able to get there with a little patience and technique. You may, however, be someone who never enjoys it, no matter how hard you try. Fortunately, there are many other options for sexy play. But if you are game to at least give it a try, here's how to approach the anus in a way that'll minimize pain and maximize success.

Using only very slight pressure, hold a toy, penis, or finger pad at the anal opening, and breathe deeply. Deep breathing will relax your whole body, including your jaw (relaxed jaw equals relaxed anus, remember?), and it'll help center you in the moment. Now, tense your anal sphincter as you breathe in and relax it on the exhale, or vice versa works, too. As you squeeze your sphincters, the anus pulls in; as you release them, the anus gently pushes out, often swallowing a small part of whatever's waiting on its doorstep in the

process. Resist the urge to forcefully push a toy, penis, or finger in. Allow the anus to open a little more with each breath, and let the toy, penis, or finger slide in ¼ inch (0.5 cm) at a time. You can even try bearing down as you relax the sphincters as though you were pushing out a BM. Oddly enough, this can actually encourage the object to slide inside. It may take up to several minutes for the object to be completely inserted.

See if you can feel your sphincters with your finger (or, if the finger belongs to someone else, ask her or him to try to feel them). Squeeze gently and notice the difference in depth and pressure that the sphincters exert on the finger. Try to notice where the external sphincter ends and the internal one begins deeper inside; there's usually only about ¼ inch (0.5 cm) of depth between them.

Once the object is at a comfortable depth, stop moving and simply let the toy, finger, or penis remain in place. Your anal sphincters are now open and are resting against it. Now most people think that this is the point at which they're supposed to start thrusting madly. Not so! It's often more pleasurable to just squeeze your sphincters, "winking" at the toy, so to speak. Notice the subtle sensations that stem from having something inside your anus. Take some more deep breaths until your sphincters are completely relaxed. If you are winking or squeezing against a penis, your partner may even ejaculate from the subtle yet powerful sensations there.

Once you're ready to try a little movement, rotate your finger or toy in circles instead of moving it in and out. Or just press gently at different points, as if you were progressing through each hour of the clock. Create vibrations by shaking your hand or by putting a vibrator in the palm of your hand to conduct the reverberations to the anus. Remember that the nerve endings most sensitive to touch are within the first inch (2.5 cm) of the anal opening (in addition, of course, to the perineal sponge and prostate, which are located deeper inside). It's a good idea to start with rotation or pressure since these movements are less likely to cause your sphincters to

squeeze from a fear of the unknown, as can happen with thrusting. And, as usual, subtle movements are often the most delightful, so pay attention to the tiniest motions.

Don't forget about the parts around your anus, either. Massage the external anal area surrounding the finger, toy, or penis while it's inside. Those external nerve endings still like being pleasured—even during penetration!

If you feel ready for it, try to insert more than one finger. You can use multiple fingers from one hand or an index finger (or more) from each hand. The great thing about using two hands is that you can alternate them for an extra-delicious sensation: One goes in while the other comes out.

When you crave the sensation of thrusting, go for it—just make sure you use enough lube. Play with speed. Each person has an ideal pace that feels perfect to her or him. Just like a massage, too-slow thrusting can be boring and too fast can be overwhelming, but there's usually a happy medium. Your ideal speed will provide exciting stimulation but won't cause you to tense up. Experiment a bit. Even if what you're doing feels amazing, try slowing down now and then to see if slower is even better. It's easy to ramp up the speed again if you prefer it faster.

FROM OUR SURVEY

It was the slowest sexual experience of my life, honestly. I was extremely slow and delicate about how I was stroking her anus and massaging her bum cheeks to make sure she was able to accept penetration. With the lube in my right hand and my left hand on her bum, I was constantly rubbing her backside, squirting lube onto my penis and her bum when it was needed, and ever so slowly moving closer, more forward and deeper into her ass. I slowly slid myself inside her, moving forward probably at about an inch every 5 minutes. She moaned, she screamed, she cried out in ecstasy. I asked her if she wanted me to take it out, and she said 'NO! Keep going. Just go slowly.' So I kept going, slowly, after finally getting my entire erection inside of her. It took a good 30 minutes for us to reach the point at which my pelvic bones were pressed against the back of her bum. It was a long process of penetration. And since it was so slow and sensual, I didn't ejaculate at all. Which is perfectly fine with me!

FROM OUR SURVEY

It actually took about a year of trying until I was able to bottom well, because I just couldn't ever relax or because I was self-conscious, and it was a frustrating cycle that actually gave me more anxiety about sex than I had had previously. But the first time I was able to successfully bottom I suddenly got why so many people really enjoy it. It didn't hurt, and it felt good, and it was fun. I thought I would be sore after but actually it was a pretty good experience. Still, it took about another 6 months to a year before I felt like I'd got the hang of it, though I still have trouble bottoming sometimes depending on who I'm with and how relaxed I feel, how big they are, or what position we're in or how much foreplay we've had beforehand.

PLAYING À DEUX

FROM OUR SURVEY

The in-stroke typically gets the prostate while the out-stroke excites the nerve endings of the two sphincters and the soft tissues of the rectal barrel.

When you're enjoying anal play with a partner, let the receiving partner—sometimes called the bottom—direct the angle, depth, and speed of penetration, especially at first. Positions that allow the bottom to move easily include squatting, kneeling, standing, kneeling on all fours, or being hunched over something like a chair, table, or bed. Once a rhythm has been established and feels good, the penetrating partner—sometimes called the top—can take over. The bottom shouldn't stop squeezing. If it feels good and is not too tiring, try squeezing as your partner thrusts in and relaxing as he or she pulls out (or vice versa). It can feel awesome to the bottom and great for your top if they have a penis inside.

Lots of folks like to combine anal play, including penetration, with other delights. Make anal a full-body experience. Play with the clitoris, vulva, penis, testicles, vagina, nipples, or breasts—or add kissing, spanking, massage, gentle touch, hair-pulling, or anything else that turns you on while you're playing with your or your partner's butt. It's all a matter of taste, though. For some people, these "extracurricular" activities are like hot fudge on an ice-cream sundae: they make anal that much sweeter. But for others, the chocolate sauce is distracting and keeps them from enjoying dessert at all. So go with whatever works best for the receiving partner. Sometimes less is more, too. For instance, simply massaging the external anal area around the inserted toy, finger, or penis can enhance the whole experience without disrupting your focus. Experimenting is the best way to find out what works for both of you.

FIVE TIPS FOR OPTIMAL INTERNAL PLAY

Focus on the golden half-inch. Remember that the nerve endings within the first ½-inch (1.3 cm) or so of the anal opening are most responsive to temperature and subtleties of touch. Go deeper and you'll only feel pressure—so adjust the type of stimulation according to the depth of penetration.

Double penetration (DP) can be exquisite for those of us with two holes. And when something's inside the vagina, the anus feels tighter—and vice versa. Plus, with DP, the perineal sponge (or prostate for trans women) gets massaged from both directions. Pure bliss! You don't need to have two penises or other large objects inside, either. A thinner, finger-size object in both holes is enough to magnify the sensations. (See chapter 10 for more on DP.)

Firm is best. It takes a pretty hard penis or toy to penetrate an anus. A softer object can work inside a vagina, but the anus is different. A less-than-hard penis or too-soft toy may buckle, especially if it's up against a nervous anus. If this happens, treat the penis and the anus to more of a warmup, or switch to a firmer (and perhaps smaller) toy—then try again.

Have a towel at the ready. Prevent E. coli infections by having a clean towel on hand to catch lube drips. Bunch up a towel and place it against the vulva of the receiving partner to catch any drips potentially containing fecal matter that may lead to an unhappy vaginal or urinary tract several days later.

Relax, and relax some more. Relaxation is absolutely key to anal play. Folks often talk about stretching the anus, but it's actually relaxation that opens the anus and rectum. You can't stretch other muscles in the body by tensing them, and the same goes for the anal sphincters and puborectal sling. If you get frustrated, take a deep breath, step back for a moment, and remember that pleasure is the goal. Don't force your anus to swallow an object. That'll only lead to pain, anal tearing, and a stressed-out butt.

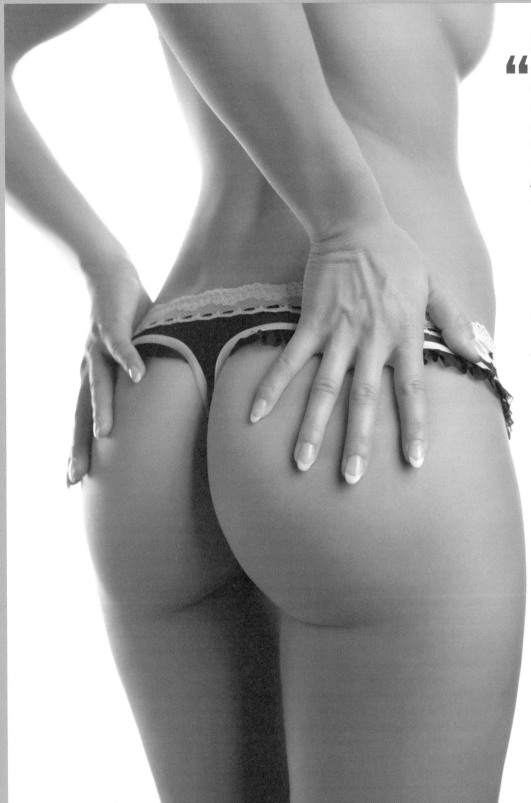

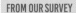

My advice: Go slow and don't worry if it doesn't work out. Try again another time; it takes practice. Do different things—rimming, fingers, toys, etc.; use different positions, different speeds, different depths; try it with different people; get in a different mood or place or context—dress up, have a bath, have a drink, plan a night to do it, do it outdoors. Have condoms and lube in convenient places. Don't worry so much about having an orgasm. Don't worry so much about staying hard or how long you last or whether you're 'clean down there.' Don't judge yourself or your partner if it doesn't work out. Talk about what feels good and what doesn't. Pay attention to your partner's reactions. Focus on how their and your body parts respond. Lose yourself in the sensation. Take breaks.

EMBRACING NEW SENSATIONS

Lots of folks tense up and freak out during the first few internal butt-play sessions because they're convinced that they're about to pass a BM. If you're the receiver, you can't see your own butt, so you can't confirm or deny those suspicions—so it becomes nearly impossible to relax into the pleasure. Counteract this fear by checking in with your partner. Then, either stop what you're doing until you're more relaxed, or take a deep breath and continue with your partner's reassurance that all is not as you fear.

You might also be uncomfortable simply because these new sensations feel unfamiliar, and our bodies often confuse newness with discomfort because they don't comprehend or recognize a feeling. Think about learning a new skill like driving: You probably struggled for a while before it became second nature. Let go of your expectations and breathe deeply. Tune in to what you feel in the present moment. Pay attention to how and where you're experiencing these new sensations. Try to stay focused. As with all kinds of sex, presence is key.

If you need to stop mid-sex when you're with a partner, that's fine. Try internal play again on your own at another time. It's often easier to allow yourself to become familiar with this new type of play without someone watching you—and without feeling like you have to prove something to someone else. (Many of us still feel the pressure to "prove" ourselves when it comes to sex, even if our rational, intellectual selves disagree.) Once your body can relax into appreciating these new sensations alone, you may be more comfortable sharing them with someone else. Like any kind of masturbation, doing it yourself can be a safe, easy way to ramp up to partner sex, since you'll be more tuned in to your own preferences and body responses.

Internal play checklist

Have all of your items on hand before you start so that you don't have to disrupt internal play mid-game to grab more tools!

- [ ] Lube for butt play, plus lube for other sensitive areas (since you might prefer a different lube for different uses)
- [ ] Gloves for hygienic fun
- [ ] Toys for the butt (and for other parts of the body, if you like!)
- [ ] Pillows for propping up legs, butts, and tummies
- [ ] Towel for catching drips of lube and juices
- [ ] Condoms for covering penises and/or toys
- [ ] Wet wipes for easy cleanup
- [ ] Towel, bucket, or sex pot (see page 148) to hold used toys
- [ ] Garbage receptacle for used condoms, gloves, tissues, or wet wipes

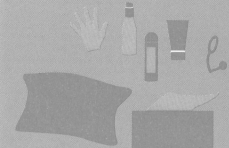

FROM OUR SURVEY

If my prostate is stimulated with direct and consistent pressure, the ejaculation that accompanies an orgasm is more copious and seems to have more velocity. The orgasm is stronger, too.

BUILD UP PLEASURE WITH BUTT PLUGS

Butt plugs are a great way to enjoy internal pleasure, either on your own or with a partner. After being inserted, they're simply left in place; there's no need to move them or play with them. What's the benefit in that? How can just leaving an object in place be pleasurable? The answer: your sphincters are special. Whenever an object is inside you, your anal sphincters are open, and that creates plenty of stimulation, no movement necessary. Even small shifts in the position of your body are magnified in the anus. In anal terms, an inch feels more like a foot. So even the slightest movements caused by breathing deeply, writhing in pleasure, or changing position will be noticeable as your anus and the toy inside it adjust ever so gently to their new positions. Some people love this style of play since it's subtle yet intensely pleasurable. You can insert a butt plug, then play with other erogenous zones—or, for extra excitement, you can wear a butt plug while you're out for a walk, at dinner with your date, or on a phone call. Any movement will draw your attention to your butt and the tantalizing possibilities butt play offers. The sensations might also make you think of your partner, so butt plugs can be a delicious way to stay connected, whether you're spending time together or apart.

And butt plugs have practical applications, too. They feel amazing, but they're also good tools for teaching your anus to accommodate toys or penises of progressively greater widths. A good plug will have a neck or valley at the base that's long and narrow enough so that the anal sphincters can rest around it without swallowing it or pushing it out. (Avoid dildos or plugs with relatively uniform widths or plugs without long necks, because your anus will push them out—or shoot them all the way across the room!—unless you hold them in place with your hand.) And make sure that anything you insert into your anus has a flared base so that it won't get "swallowed" by the rectum. There's a situation that has unenviable consequences, to put it mildly.

Once the dildo or plug is securely in place, by all means focus on whatever other activities bring you pleasure, like penis, clit, or vaginal play; nipple stimulation; toe sucking; kissing; spanking—whatever feels awesome to you. Then, after it's been in place for a few minutes, the plug or dildo can usually be taken out slowly, and a slightly wider toy or penis can be inserted without discomfort. The other advantage of a butt plug (or a dildo held in place; no thrusting) is that the lack of in-and-out movement truly allows the sphincters to relax around the toy. Don't get me wrong: thrusting can feel incredible. But when a dildo, finger(s), or penis/outie thrusts in and out, the anus can't relax as much because the sphincters are more engaged and alert. And this means that the anus will become fatigued more quickly and may not respond as positively to a toy of a larger width. (Think of it

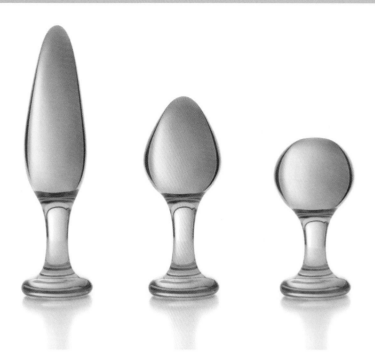

FROM OUR SURVEY

Sometimes anal stimulation and pressure on the prostate can make it difficult to achieve an erection, but if I'm already hard and I'm close to coming before the prostate play starts, I can actually get harder.

like this: Wouldn't you be more open to a workout at the gym if you'd had some rest beforehand—instead of, say, after a strenuous bike ride?)

Speaking of width, when it comes to internal anal play, the most critical consideration for most people is the width of the toy or penis they plan to insert. As I often tell my customers, make sure that your eyes aren't wider than your butt! What might look like a handsome, satisfying toy might turn out to be hard to swallow and could end up being more painful than pleasurable. Also, I generally advise beginners not to insert anything that's wider than what comes out of the anus—that is, a BM—since your body is already used to accommodating things of that size. Increasing that width requires more patience and time.

That said, length does play a part when it comes to butt plugs. A plug or toy that's long enough to hit the prostate or the perineal

sponge definitely opens up more possibilities. For most folks, a toy that's 6 inches (15 cm) long should be sufficient—and with a toy of this length, there's no danger of entering the colon (it has a complicated angle that's usually too much for beginners to contend with). If you're an advanced anal player and you like to use extra-long dildos or arms, be sure to go slowly and to pay attention to the body's signals so that you won't cause damage to the digestive tract.

Finally, this is not a time to be goal-oriented. You won't necessarily feel more pleasure by accommodating a larger toy. In the same way that eating a huge meal isn't enjoyable once your stomach is full, don't try to force yourself to take in something that's too big for you. It'll lead to disappointment or pain—or both. Respect your limits for the day. Even if you were able to take a 2-inch (5-cm) toy last week, your body might not enjoy it this time around. Build up toy size gradually, and stop when it feels just right.

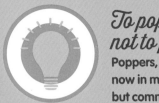

To pop or not to pop

Poppers, illegal now in many places but commonly used for anal sex, are made of alkyl nitrite. It is packaged under many names, such as leather cleaner. Inhaling this chemical causes vasodilation (dilation of the blood vessels). The short-term (up to 90 seconds) effect is that of muscle relaxation. Many folks use poppers because they find that they can relax into anal play much more easily and have heightened orgasms. Speculation on the chemical's negative effects are inconclusive; however, it has led to short-term effects such as headaches, impotence, and fainting. Newer varieties of poppers are reported to be more harmful, with effects such as permanent memory impairment and "sudden sniffing death," aka arrhythmia. I do not advise using them. Lots of folks have awesome popper-free anal sex!

FROM OUR SURVEY

" After I have an orgasm with toys, retrieving them can be a problem. With their bulbous heads, taking them out is uncomfortable, almost painful. After coming, my ass is interested in returning to its normal state—and that isn't loose enough to pass these sizable toys easily. "

PRESENCE AND COMMUNICATION DURING INTERNAL PLAY

As humans, we communicate with one another in so many ways: body language, tone, word choice, breathing, body movement, and uncensored physical reactions. If you're the top, tune in to the many ways in which your partner is communicating with you. Even if she or he is actually saying yes to what you're doing, the body may express its reluctance through shallow breathing, tension in the anus and body, word flow, and vocal pitch. Check in with your partner if you feel that her or his physical and verbal reactions seem dissonant.

Also, it's important to remain aware of your own process and needs. For example, if you don't feel confident, your touch may feel tentative and not as pleasurable to your partner. Notice if you find yourself moving your hands or a toy more quickly. This is often a sign that you're nervous and unsure of what to do next. When this happens, stop for a moment and check in with yourself and your partner. Take some deep breaths and keep going only when you feel more confident. If you don't know what your partner wants, ask her or him. And if your partner seems a little less than fully engaged as the bottom, reassure her or him with plenty of positive feedback. Often, a little encouragement is all it takes.

When internal play is finished, it can feel really comforting and tender to keep a hand on the outside of the anus after you pull out whatever was inside. The anus closes gradually, and it can feel lonely and abandoned if the intensity suddenly drops from ninety-nine to zero, especially after an intense session. Lay your fingers across the anus, within the crack of the butt cheeks. This soothing sensation can really be the icing on the proverbial cake. Simply hold your fingers in place without moving them while you kiss, debrief, or fall asleep. These small attentions to detail are what heighten the experience—leaving you eager to try it all over again soon.

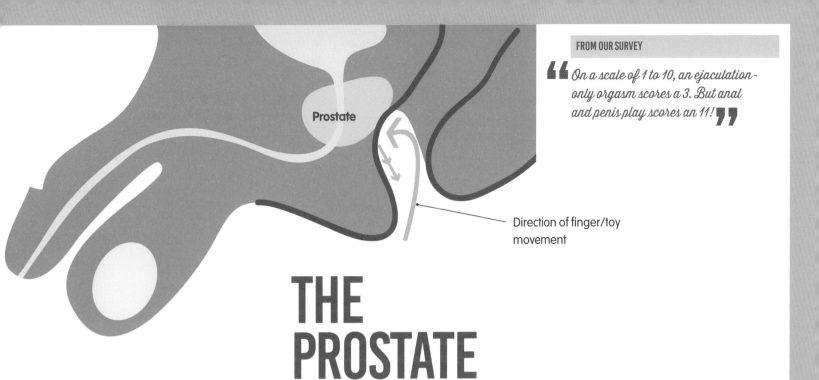

Prostate

Direction of finger/toy movement

FROM OUR SURVEY

On a scale of 1 to 10, an ejaculation-only orgasm scores a 3. But anal and penis play scores an 11!

THE PROSTATE

The prostate is a gland in the male reproductive system that produces some of the milky fluid that combines with sperm to form ejaculate. It can be stimulated through the rectum, and this stimulation, according to lots of prostate players, results in eye-popping, full-body orgasms.

That said, as you can see from Jon's story on the next page, we all respond differently to various types of pleasure. For instance, some people love nipple stimulation; others, not so much. Clitoral play—the Holy Grail of pleasure for lots of women—can be too intense for some folks, while others just don't find it that interesting. In general, most penises enjoy being pleasured—but when penis play is combined with anal play, responses can vary. In some cases, that may include the loss of an erection. This doesn't mean that the penis's owner doesn't enjoy butt play, though. It might simply mean that the sensation is different or unfamiliar or that all the focus has shifted to the anal area. Some people like to have both areas pleasured individually, or simultaneously—or through a certain sequence of stimulation. Some folks always ejaculate from prostate play, and others rarely do. One thing's for sure: each prostate is as unique as its owner! If you have a prostate—or if your partner has one—it might be worth exploring the pleasure it can offer.

Locating the prostate

Where *is* the prostate, anyway? It lies below the bladder and next to the rectum (the urethra passes through it), so it's not located in the rectum, per se, but you can feel it through the rectum's front wall. Here's how to find it. Insert a toy or finger (or penis, if you like, but they tend to be a little wide for beginners) about 2–4 inches (5–10 cm) inside and angle it toward the belly button. The prostate feels like a cherry tomato–sized bump with a dip or valley all around it, and it's squishy to the touch, like the tip of a nose.

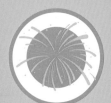

Prostate stimulation and orgasm

Prostate stimulation is the little secret that's gaining traction as a delicious, exotic new item on our sex menus. It might not suit everyone's palate, but those who do like prostate pleasure are eager to order it up again and again—and again.

According to prevailing stereotypes, if you have a penis, then you want all sexual stimulation to be focused on it—period. Now, don't get me wrong: penis stimulation is fantastic, and it's easy to understand how the phallus fallacy took root. But it isn't the only erogenous zone. The prostate can change sex entirely.

When the penis is touched, licked, or engulfed, the sensation is very localized: it's confined to that stretch of skin. Sure, the pleasure radiates from there throughout the body, but the focal point of fun is primarily the head and secondarily the shaft. It's very direct, very easy to manipulate, and it's fairly predictable. Let's not go so far as to say all penises like the same thing, but some commonplace moves will almost always excite a penis.

Conversely, prostate stimulation is more like a circular journey. Arriving at your destination doesn't complete the trip; arriving just means the beginning of the next act.

Remember how I described penis stimulation as localized? Well, prostate touch is both hyper-localized and all encompassing. The first time someone touched my prostate, I saw stars and lightning bolts. The sensation can be so intense that it radiates throughout the body, weakening limbs and creating tremendous tactile response.

And that's just touch. Can you imagine a prostate-induced orgasm?

To be fair, I've only ever had two prostate-only orgasms. They can happen, but they take work. I rarely have the patience to wait that long, so I involve my penis in the fun before I get off. But if you *can* wait, the orgasm is unlike any other. For me, it wasn't just a wonderful physical experience; it was also a tremendous exploration of my sexuality. To see ejaculate emerge from your cock—without having touched it—is a remarkable visual after years of direct physical contact. (All of this is provided you can keep your eyes open during the hard, deep orgasm you are experiencing!)

There are distinct similarities and differences between penis and prostate orgasms. Penis orgasms feel lighter, more like you're emitting something into the world. On the other hand, prostate orgasms feel more like you're gasping and grasping for more inside you. It is heavy and dense and full of pleasure. Now, combine the two, and you might never want to get out of bed ever again!

—From Jon Pressick, broadcaster and sex expert

FROM OUR SURVEY

"I'm female, and my male partner loves prostate stimulation. I love massaging his prostate. He gets so incredibly turned on, and so quickly. He would ejaculate from prostate stimulation, but he usually stops himself because he wants to continue playing."

On EmptyClosets.com, one expert describes it this way: "Place the tip of your tongue in your cheek between your molars. Then use your index [finger] to rub the cheek over the tip of your tongue—that's close to what it will feel like. It's like a soft 'bump' that is a little firmer than the tissue around it."

Often, it's easier to find when you're aroused since arousal causes the prostate to fill with fluid, so try looking for it after a little genital play. Usually, the owner of the prostate will know pretty quickly when it's been touched and may even ejaculate right after it's been stimulated. Some folks know they've found it when they feel like they have to pee. This makes perfect sense, because the prostate is located under the bladder and because the urethra passes through the prostate. If you or your partner find this feeling uncomfortable, focus on the pleasure and take plenty of deep

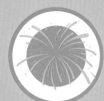

Trans women, G-spots, and prostates

When folks talk about the G-spot, they're often referring to two separate anatomical features: the erectile tissue that surrounds the urethra and the Skene's gland. The Skene's gland is, essentially, the same thing as the prostate, and it's sometimes called "the female prostate"—probably because of prevailing gender anxieties, which tend to reinforce the differences between the sexes instead of the similarities.

Now, for a lot of folks, this might be purely academic, but it can be very meaningful for trans women. Although it depends upon your surgeon's technique, if you've had vaginoplasty (surgery where a vagina is created), quite often the vaginal canal is placed just in front of the prostate, with that bundle of erectile tissue surrounding the urethra just on the other side. That's right: trans women can have both P-spots *and* G-spots. What's more, it also means that the prostate can be stimulated from two sides—vaginally and anally—at the same time. Imagine the possibilities!

—*From Tobi Hill-Meyer, sex-positive activist, writer, and porn-maker*

FROM OUR SURVEY

" I have full anal orgasms involving the prostate, where sometimes I ejaculate. Those orgasms are very intense, and my ass feels totally awesome, but the ejaculation isn't the same familiar pleasure. It's mostly just wet. "

breaths. This often dissipates the discomfort and reveals the intense sensations that lie beneath it.

The first time you go exploring, you might not feel anything right away. Don't despair. You may just need to become a little more aroused or play with different kinds of touch until your body responds. If butt play in general is new to you, you might need to get used to the new sensations in your sphincters and rectum before you can tune in to what's going on with your prostate.

Fingers are the most discerning way of pleasuring the prostate. Toys are great, too, since they basically act as arm extensions, helping you to reach the prostate more easily—but with toys, it's harder to tell whether you're hitting the right spot. The fingers of a giver are more accurate since

they can feel their way around. (If you're the giver, make sure to use the pads of your fingers rather than the tips to avoid sharp nails poking sensitive rectal tissue.) In either case, for solo play, you can either reach between your legs or reach around from behind your back. Reaching between your legs can require your wrist to bend at a tough angle, so this might not be the best option, depending on your flexibility and tummy size. Reaching around from behind can be challenging, too, since it's harder to apply pressure to the front wall of the rectum, where the prostate is located. Using a thumb instead of a finger can help with the angle—if your thumbs are long enough to reach the prostate, that is. It all depends on your individual anatomy, so do a little solo exploration to see which positions work best for you and your prostate!

Can massage promote a healthy prostate?

Ah, massage. It feels great just about anywhere on your body, doesn't it? And the prostate is no exception. But while the benefits of general massage are well-known today, to date there are no known studies that have investigated the health benefits of prostate massage. Before the advent of antibiotics, though, medical professionals recommended prostate massage, which seemed to alleviate prostatitis, or infection of the prostate gland. It was believed to assist in flushing bacteria and fluid from the prostate. Now that we have antibiotics to help fight infections, prostate massage has fallen out of fashion—although many folks argue that its health benefits still exist. Like any other type of massage, prostate massage stimulates circulation and the movement of stagnant fluids. And with our sedentary twenty-first-century lifestyles, that can only be a good thing. Some people even claim that promoting vigorous circulation of blood and other fluids in this way can prevent prostate-related problems, such as cancer.

But why bother with prostate massage at all? Isn't ejaculation enough to get those fluids moving, and if so, shouldn't you just masturbate and/or have sex regularly? The answer is that regular ejaculation also shifts stagnant energy and fluids and promotes circulation—but prostate-focused stimulation can flush out the prostate more thoroughly. Plus, getting to know your prostate is a good thing. That way, you'll notice small changes in it before your annual checkup rolls around, and you can look into these changes before any problems develop. And it feels great, to boot! So there's really no reason *not* to get buddy-buddy with your prostate.

FROM OUR SURVEY

" Prostate orgasms are electric. I've only experienced a few, and only one with ejaculation. "

How to milk the prostate

The prostate feels like a ripe tomato with a valley down its middle. That valley is how fluid drains from it. According to *The Ultimate Guide to Prostate Pleasure* by Charlie Glickman, Ph.D., and Aislinn Emirzian, the best way to drain the prostate of most of its fluid is to think of it as a clock. Start at nine o'clock, and apply gentle pressure as you move your finger to the middle of the clock where the hands are anchored. Then move your finger to three o'clock—and back to the middle again. Next, move your finger to two o'clock. Apply pressure toward ten o'clock, but stop in the middle. Then start at ten o'clock, and move your finger toward two o'clock. Repeat, moving from one o'clock to eleven, and from eleven back to one. Then head south: begin at four o'clock and move your finger toward eight, then back toward four; move from five toward seven and back again, always stopping in the middle, and always lifting your finger and returning to the side.

FROM OUR SURVEY

" Prostate orgasms are certainly the most intense. Sometimes I just like being fucked because it can feel euphoric for long sessions and I'm not sure I really have an orgasm . . . Everything just feels incredible. "

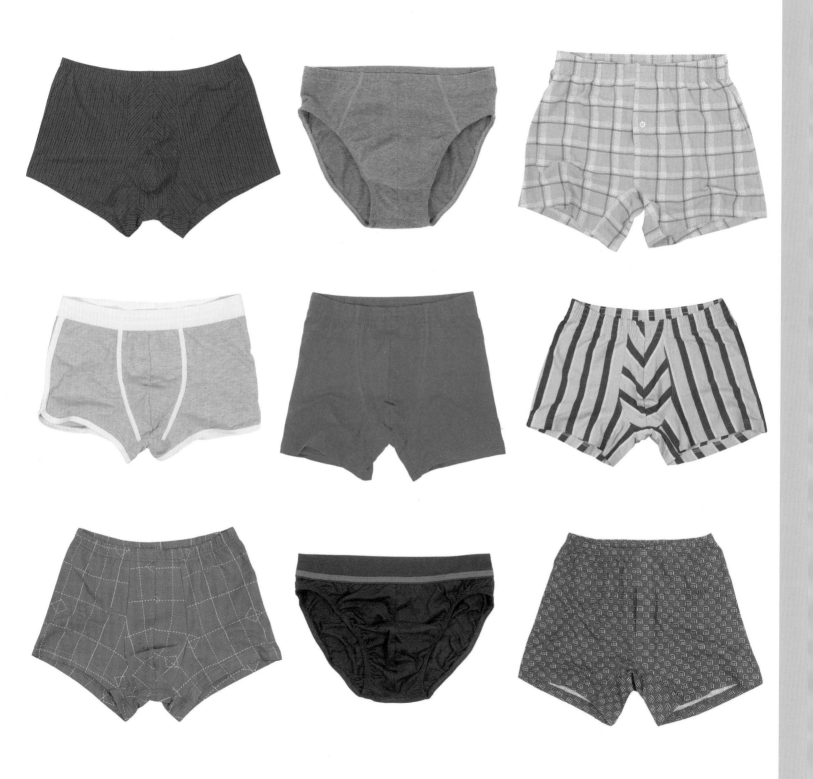

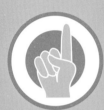

Exploring your prostate

Relax, breathe, and slow down. Then, glide the tip of the finger in to the first knuckle. Make a little stirring motion. Try a little pulse, like a tiny pump, and then try quicker vibrations. Move the fingertip up and down, then side to side. Honor the four directions. Have the receiver clench the butthole. Try a clench that closes on the inhale and releases on the outbreath. Do this slowly, and then more quickly.

Add more lube. See if you can slide the finger in farther, perhaps up to the second knuckle. Using the finger, repeat the stirring motion, vibrations, and side-to-side and up-and-down motions. These movements will open the walls of the sphincter, allowing the inner anus to open up.

When you find the prostate, do a little wave with your fingertip. Circle the orb in one direction, then the other. Pump a little, tap a little, flick a little; strumming, plucking and dabbing can also increase sensation. (Vibrations are always good!) Check with your partner to see whether these sensations are too much or too little, and adjust accordingly.

For a little more action at the prostate, try some slide-and-glide. Slide in, using one finger, two fingers, or a toy. Try nudging and dabbing at the prostate. If you have two fingers inside, try twiddling them together as you bump the center of the prostate, or slide them around the edges of the orb. "Scissor" your fingers by moving them apart slightly and then bringing them together. Remember that with a toy, subtle motions are accentuated and amplified since the toy is not nearly as sensitive as a finger or two. Slow, sensual motions will bring a smoother response. Go a little farther, a little faster, a little harder as the receiver relaxes and opens. Use lots of lube, relax, breathe, let go, and have a delightful time.

—From Phillip Coupal, counsellor, coach, and bodywork practitioner (www.phillipcoupal.com)

The ground rules of prostate play

Warm up. Touching the prostate is like touching the penis or clitoris: it can be pretty intense, and it can feel unpleasant when touched quickly or forcefully, so you'll want to move toward it slowly. Give yourself plenty of time, and don't rush.

No speeding. Play around with the speed of your finger or toy, or your thrusting movement. Faster is rarely better since most people tense up when faced with stimulation—prostate or otherwise—that's too fast. And if this kind of play is new to you, your sphincters will be surprised and confused if you move too quickly. For most people, a slow or medium pace works best. Experiment by using different techniques at different speeds and levels of arousal.

Stick with it. Once you've found your ideal speed, stay there. Regardless of our equipment—clitoris, penis, and/or prostate—we often need rhythmic movement in order to orgasm. And sometimes it takes a minute or two for the rhythm to register in our nerve receptors and brains. Give the rhythm time to gain momentum, and don't expect instant fireworks, even if what you're doing already feels amazing.

More techniques for prostate pleasure

If you've tried the prostate-milking techniques on page 84, move on to these techniques for a little extra exploration.

The Doorbell. Press on the prostate with the pad of your finger, as if you were ringing a doorbell again and again.

The Windshield Wiper. Move your finger back and forth over the same area. Shift from windshield-wiping at the midway point (three to nine o'clock and back) to the upper part (eleven to one o'clock) or the lower part (eight to four o'clock). If you insert two fingers, you can hold them side by side as you move them, or you can place one finger at each side of the prostate, moving them so that they meet back in the middle—like making a peace sign with your hand and opening and closing the *V*.

Circles. Make tiny circles that focus on each number on the clock—or make large circles around the perimeter of the prostate "clock."

Vibration. Vibrate your finger while it's inside, or hold a vibrator against your hand to conduct the vibration. Of course, you can also insert a vibrator with a flared base (see chapter 8).

Come Hither. G-spots often like this technique, too. Make a "come hither" motion with one or more fingers while you move your fingers up and down the prostate. Or spread two fingers into a peace sign, and make the tips travel down the sides of the prostate.

FROM OUR SURVEY

"Prostate play can change the focus of my sensations from my penis to my ass. If I'm only playing with my ass and not my penis, I may only get partially hard. But coming from penile stimulation plus ass play generally feels better. The orgasm is 'bigger' and more intense, and while I haven't exactly measured it, I also feel like I cum more."

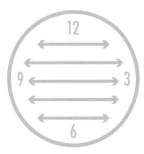

The Windshield Wiper

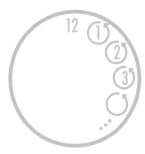

Circles

FROM OUR SURVEY

It was extremely sensitive, and I could feel the fingers push on a part of my body that had never been touched before. . . . It kinda felt like someone was tickling underneath my bladder with a hand that started from inside my body.

In Joseph Kramer's DVD *Anal Massage for Lovers*, there is an amazing prostate massage scene that offers much sage advice. One suggestion is to insert two fingers into the prostate and place your thumb on one side and ring finger to the other side of the testicles to massage the base of the penis. You can also anchor your partner's whole body with your hand and rotate his torso via the movement of your whole hand for an extra-delicious, full-body rocking sensation.

Prostate-play orgasms

No two orgasms are alike, either. So before you play, you'll want to adjust your expectations. If you anticipate the sensations in advance or compare them to other kinds of pleasure you've experienced, you might end up missing the incredible, toe-curling feelings that you didn't expect at all. Be aware of your body's responses, and accept them as they come (no pun intended!). Some people

orgasm from prostate play alone, but many others don't orgasm in this way at all, or need additional genital play to climax. Many people find that prostate-play orgasms release more fluid than "regular" ones; others love the way their arousal is less focused during prostate pleasure, which can mean longer, more intense sensations whether you orgasm or not. And whereas most of the time, the "point of no return" that precedes ejaculation is super-pleasurable but quite short, with prostate play, you can ride that wave of arousal for much longer before going over the edge. What's not to like?

Finally, with all of your freshly flowing juices and your reinvigorated blood circulation, you might feel a little sore afterward, so go easy the first time you try prostate play. Don't start out with a marathon session; overstimulation will only tire out your muscles (and your sweet spots, too!).

Rocketships, fireworks, intense, and **explosive**—these are just some of the adjectives people use to describe their orgasms as a result of prostate play—and even folks who don't orgasm from it often find it uniquely pleasurable. The sensations that arise from prostate play tend to be deeper, more full-bodied, longer, or more intense than those that arise from cock play. Of course, since no two people are alike, this isn't true for everyone.

Multiple orgasms?

People of all genders can experience multiple orgasms from many types of play, and prostate play is one way of getting there. Orgasm and ejaculation are two separate events, but they're often experienced as one and the same. That's because, for most people with prostates, the two events happen within about 1 second of each other. After experiencing this sensation hundreds (or thousands) of times, it starts to feel like a single event. Some men and trans women learn how to separate their orgasms from ejaculation in order to achieve multiple orgasms. While ejaculation—that is, the emission of fluid—saps energy, causes erections to subside, and makes you sleepy, orgasms are contractions of the pelvic floor muscles, and they can happen over and over again. Learning how to have nonejaculatory orgasms can extend pleasure. To learn more about this technique, see Mantak Chia's *The Multi-Orgasmic Man: The Sexual Secrets That Every Man Should Know.*

But you won't know whether prostate play is for you until you try it—so consider giving it a try and deciding for yourself. Whether it works for you or not, a thirst for exploration is what keeps sex fun, interesting, and fulfilling. Great communication with your partner doesn't hurt, either—and chapter 6 will show you how to get there.

FROM OUR SURVEY

" *I like anal sex because it's a whole area of sensation that also allows for more intense orgasms. I've also had a purely anal orgasm or two, and I really enjoyed those— particularly since they allow for multiple orgasms and are just a different, more 'whole-body' feeling. Undoubtedly there is also a bit of the thrill of the abjectness of it all. As a male-bodied person, it's also important for me because I like to be the fuckee rather than simply the fucker.* "

Chapter 6
COMMUNICATION:
THE KEY TO HOT, SEXY, BONDED ANAL PLAY

We all know how important communication is to a healthy relationship. And you might be perfectly comfortable telling your partner or partners where you want to meet for dinner, how you'd like to celebrate your birthday, that it's her turn to clean the bathroom, or that you want him to take charge of the vacation plans this year. But somehow, when it comes to sex, it's not always that easy. Communication—or the lack thereof—is the most significant determinant in the quality of your sex life, but if you've ever given instructions to a partner about how you want to be pleasured, you may have already realized that what you say and what your partner does in response don't always match up. There are a couple reasons for that. First of all, language is fluid, and your experiences, preferences, and assumptions can affect how you interpret another person's request. Plus, you may have held back from articulating your desires to your partner from a fear of rejection or judgment, or from plain old awkwardness or embarrassment. That's completely understandable. It can be difficult to bring up your true desires and reveal your authentic self, especially when there's a lot at stake. But you *can* have a frank, open conversation with your partner about sex, including the possibility of anal play. This chapter will show you how to organize your thoughts before you bring up the subject of anal with your partner; how to frame the discussion in a positive, nonjudgmental way; what to do if your partner just isn't into it; and lots more.

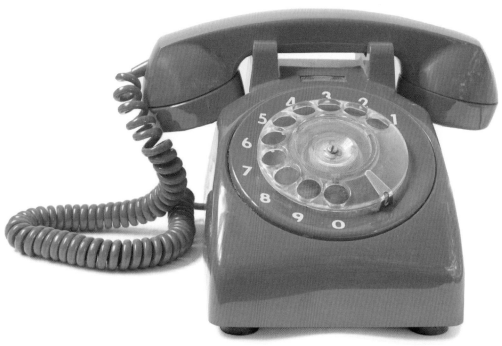

BE INTROSPECTIVE

FROM OUR SURVEY

" *This one time, I was with my partner in a bathhouse, and he was playing with another guy and had a finger or two up his bum. When the finger came out, his bowels relaxed unintentionally and he pooped on the floor. The dude immediately bolted, and we looked at each other and just kinda shrugged and went to go shower. But actually, when we were packing up to go later, he came back around, and we were all chatting and it was totally whatever. Shit happens.* "

Before you approach your partner, take a step back for a moment. Take a deep breath, and remind yourself that your desires, preferences, and fantasies are both valid and important. Remember that you have the right to decide how you want to enjoy sexual pleasure and to explore your sexuality. And regardless of your partner's reaction (which is just as likely to be positive as it is to be negative, by the way), your desire to explore anal sex is your own, and it deserves respect.

Then give yourself a break. Anal sex isn't the only topic that's tough to discuss. When it comes to sex, it can be hard to bring up *anything* new—the idea of using sex toys, trying kinky sex, experimenting with butt play, and even introducing the use of lubricant can all lead to awkward conversations. So before you initiate a conversation about anal sex, think about why you want to have sex with

your partner in general (apart from anal sex specifically). Your motivations might include building intimacy or connection, having fun, finding new erogenous zones, enjoying exploration and adventure, expressing your love for her or him, or other reasons that are important to you. It's a good idea to do this in advance because it'll help you articulate to your partner your reasons for wanting to explore this activity together.

After you consider your reasons for wanting to have sex with your partner in general, reflect on why you want to try anal sex in particular. Does it offer you an opportunity to penetrate or be penetrated for the first time? Is it because you want to try a different kind of sex? Do you get turned on by the idea of experimenting with something that's "taboo"? Are you hoping to discover new levels of pleasure? Will it give you a chance to take control or to allow yourself to be vulnerable? Or do you simply think it might be fun? All of these are perfectly valid.

Especially if you think your partner might be reluctant to try anal sex, it's a good idea do your homework ahead of time. Before you bring up the topic with your partner, be prepared to address the common fears and concerns surrounding anal sex, including issues of cleanliness, safety, and pain. That way, it'll be easier for you to gently and respectfully address your partner's reservations and to help her or him understand the facts. (Also, feel free to extol the virtues of anal play. The potential for intense pleasure, increased intimacy, and even enhanced anal health might encourage your partner to consider it, and a great sales pitch can't do any harm!)

Ten ground rules for talking about sex with your partner

1. Accept that conversations about sex are healthy and necessary. They can be hard to initiate, but an honest discussion can lead to feeling closer, getting what you want, and knowing how to better satisfy your partner.

2. Enter the conversation with an open mind and with a willingness to understand your partner's efforts and positive intentions. Be caring and constructive in your approach. Your goal is to strengthen your relationship.

3. If there is a problem or concern, try to understand the real issue. If you unearth something, dig deeper in case there is a bigger issue hidden.

4. Be sure to acknowledge your love and admiration for your partner. Reassure him or her of your commitment and care, whether he or she was the one who brought up a tough subject or you were the initiator.

5. Express your own needs and desires for the relationship. Use "I" statements. Try to bring to possible resolutions to the discussion if something is not working.

6. Be honest, clear, and sincere. Ask for what you need in order to feel comfortable sharing your personal thoughts and wishes.

7. Listen carefully and clarify. Don't interrupt. Repeat back what your partner said to be sure you really understand what he or she is saying.

8. Be patient and take breaks if necessary. Allow the process the time that it needs for everyone to feel heard and understood and to express his or her perspective. Revisit the conversation at a later date if necessary.

9. Remain present. Lock the door if you need to, and avoid other distractions. Notice what triggers you or makes you feel defensive, take a breath, and step back. You want to listen to what your partner is actually saying, not just what your own head is telling you.

10. Check out any assumptions. Oftentimes what you assume is true isn't true at all. The more you assume, the further you may go down the wrong path.

FROM OUR SURVEY

" *With a new partner, I usually bring up anal sex outside of the bedroom in general getting-to-know-you conversation.* "

HOW TO TALK TO YOUR PARTNER ABOUT ANAL SEX

When it comes to talking about sex, how you approach the conversation is just as important as what you say during it. Here are a few things to keep in mind when you're planning a frank discussion about sex. . . .

Watch your timing

Make sure you've cleared the air of any outstanding (non-sex-related) issues, like your frustration over chores that've been left undone, the fact that you haven't gotten to spend enough quality time together recently, or how you hate that your partner is always, *always* late for rendezvous. Once issues like these have been resolved, make sure that you've let go of lingering resentments or anger. The last thing you want to do is to mix up a conversation about anal sex with a back-and-forth over who left that huge stack of dirty dishes in the sink.

Then, identify an opportune moment for an intimate talk. Here's when *not* to instigate a discussion about sex: right before your parents arrive for dinner, during an argument, or when you're actually in the middle of having sex. Instead, choose a moment in which neither one of you is in a hurry and when you're both feeling relatively relaxed—perhaps when you're cuddling, sharing a meal, or just chatting after a satisfying sex romp. Alternatively, think about setting aside some time each week (or every two weeks, or each month) to check in with your partner on how things are going—financially, emotionally, or erotically. "Taking the temperature" of a relationship in this way helps ensure that you're both happy with things the way they are, and that you're both

comfortable with where you're going. And it's an ideal time to talk about your sexual desires and fantasies—including anal play. Checking in with each other regularly prevents resentment from building up in either or both of you and lets you voice your dissatisfaction before a major blow-up takes place.

Use simple communication techniques to start

Begin by talking about yourself. How are you feeling in the moment? Name the emotions—such as awkwardness, fear, anxiety, excitement—that arise from bringing up a new topic or from talking about your sex life at all. As you broach the topic, take responsibility for and talk about your own feelings and desires, limitations, and fears. Even if you are feeling erotically uninspired in this relationship, take ownership in the ways that you contribute to or enable this pattern. Nobody wants to feel blamed, so try not to focus solely on what's wrong or on what isn't working. Instead, open the discussion by telling your partner what you love about your sex life, since a positive approach will make her or him feel comfortable, open, and ready to pay close attention to what you're saying.

A more playful (but no less informative!) way to kick off a discussion about sex is to play a communication game called Three Oranges and a Lemon. In it, each person tells the other three things that they love about their erotic life together, plus one thing that they'd like to do differently. For example, you might say:

"I love that you like to surprise me with new toys and sexy clothes."

"I love how you throw me up against the wall and kiss me deeply."

"I love the way you give me oral sex until I come."

"And I'd love to try anal play—on both of us," or "And I'd love to add some variety to our repertoire, like anal pleasure," or "I'm curious about prostate play"—whatever it is that you'd like to try.

Of course, sometimes we find ourselves too nervous to initiate conversations like these because we're afraid of how our partners will interpret them. But a little prep work before the convo starts can go a long way.

Sex and relationship expert Reid Mihalko has developed a simple process for helping people organize their ideas and prepare what they want to articulate to their partners in a way that will encourage acceptance and understanding. Here's his formula for broaching difficult subjects:

Use the following statements as platforms for brainstorming. Think of as many different answers for each you as you can.

A. What I'm not saying to my partner is
_____.

(e.g., "I'd like to try anal sex," "I'd love to explore my/your/our prostate(s)," "Sometimes I want to lick your butthole when I'm going down on you.")

B. What I'm afraid might happen if I say it is
_____.

(e.g., "You'll think I'm a pervert," "You'll think differently of me," "You'll think I'm weak." Remember, you're brainstorming! Your list can be as long as you want it to be.)

C. What I'd like to make happen by saying this is
_____.

(e.g., "We'll keep our sex life interesting," "We'll explore something new together," "We'll grow closer," "I'll allow myself to be vulnerable with my partner." Write down all the positive things that come to mind!)

Then, when you're ready to have the conversation, you'll rearrange this formula a bit. You'll start with B, or your fears; followed by C, your desires; and finish with A, the statement that makes you feel a bit shaky. To the right is an example of how the conversation might take shape.

Dear [partner's name or nickname],

There's something I want to talk to you about, and I'm having a hard time with it because I'm afraid the following might happen: [explain the answers you came up with from the B statement to the left].

The reason I want to tell you about this is that, by doing so, I hope that: [the answers you came up with from the C statement to the left].

So, what I'd like to tell you is: [the answers you came up with from the A statement to the left].

Thank you for listening. Do you want to share anything with me? And do you have any questions about what I mean, or about anal play in general?

Sample Letter

FROM OUR SURVEY

The only time when I was the one to bring up anal sex first was in the context of this book! I have always really wanted anal sex play—in theory—but I've never been brave enough to actually go there. But I fantasize and verbalize about anal play a lot in my fantasies and in kinky talk during mutual masturbation—so when the opportunity came up to contribute to this book, experiment with new toys, and get some guidance through Carlyle's videos, I jumped at the chance to finally explore all the pleasures that anal play could provide.

With this approach, you're being up-front about the fact that you're nervous or anxious about what you want to say, you're being positive and proactive, and you're giving your partner a chance to respond and to voice her or his own thoughts and concerns. So try it out! You can even download a worksheet to help you organize your thoughts at www.reidaboutsex.com.

Give it some space

Once you've broached the subject of anal sex with your partner, give her or him some time to sit with his or her thoughts. Your partner may surprise you with a super-positive reaction, like "I thought you'd never ask!"—or it might take a little while for her or him to process the idea and figure out how to feel

about it. After your conversation, leave your partner with some helpful resources (like this book, and flag the pages you think are especially relevant!), with websites that sell toys you'd like to try, or with information on safer sex. Give your partner the space to do a little research and, perhaps, to talk to trusted friends. Check in with your partner again in a week or two, asking how her or his feelings have evolved. Be prepared to learn that your partner is not interested in anal play—but remember that regardless of your partner's response, you'll always be able to play with your own butt! It may not be your number-one fantasy, but you can still do plenty of exploring on your own. And you might even find ways to self-pleasure your butt during partner sex. Of course, if what you really want to do is

penetrate your partner, anal play simply may not be in the cards if your partner isn't up for it. In that case, try this: Visualize your anal fantasy in full, and break it down into parts. Without pressuring your partner, share your fantasy with her or him and try to discern whether there's a midway point or a beginning strategy. For instance, you might agree that external play is okay, but not internal play. Or perhaps using toys for penetration is okay, but a penis isn't. See if there's a way to compromise so that you can fulfill some of your desires without violating your partner's boundaries.

The yes/no/maybe game

Sometimes it's helpful to break down sex acts into distinct options instead of thinking of them in more general terms. After all, the phrase *anal sex* might seem more than a little overwhelming. That's where the Yes/No/Maybe game comes in. Fill out the chart with your preferences for each activity, and invite your partner to do the same. This might seem a bit too much like school at first, but trust me, it's worth it. You may find that you and your partner share more common ground than you imagined.

Put a check in the appropriate box for each line, and if you can, comment on your response in the Specifics box to help explain your reasons for your choice. For instance, you might write, "Tried it once, but I'd had a few drinks" or "It hurt," or "I didn't like it, but I didn't know what I was doing," or even "Open to it, but need more information on how to do it safely." It's also a great way to organize your thoughts and to figure out what you'd like to try and what you'd rather avoid. You can fill out one form for receiving the techniques and another for trying them on your partner. Or you could fill it in with blue ink for receiving (bottoming) and red for giving (topping).

Dealing with disappointment

Learning that your partner isn't into anal sex may be tough for you to hear, but if that's the case, it's important that you honor her or his choice. Your partner's desires, choices, and boundaries deserve respect in the same way that yours do. Be as nonjudgmental as possible, and remember that a person's individual preferences do not mean that she or he is a "pervert" or a "prude" and that preferences may change over time. Ultimately, sex is about choice free from pressure or unfair consequences. Different desires are simply a fact of life, and that's not only true for sexual activities. Financial priorities, living arrangements, and travel plans all require compromise!

FROM OUR SURVEY

I asked my partner if he had ever tried anal play. He just looked at me. Then he asked, 'Do you mean . . . in the ass?' He had never tried it, and he hadn't been with a woman who had ever brought it up before. He didn't realize how much he would love it, or that it would become a regular feature in our sexual repertoire.

ANAL SEX QUESTIONNAIRE

Activity	Yes	No	Maybe	Specifics (details, considerations, limitations)
Finger on outside				
Vibrator on outside				
Tongue on outside				
Finger(s) inside				
Vibrator inside				
Tongue inside				
Prostate finger play				
Prostate toy play				
Butt plug (or something stationary) on inside				
Dildo moving inside				
Penis inside				
Anal play in combination with penis/clit/vagina/ nipple play				
Solo anal play during other kinds of sex				

ONE, TWO, CONSENT: GO!

Once you and your partner have agreed that you're both up for anal play, both of you need to be clear about your rules and boundaries. Start by playing the Yes/No/Maybe game together. Talk about your feelings. What turns you on? What makes you nervous or fearful? Be open about your previous experiences and about what worked for you and what didn't. Be specific and talk about as many aspects of your (real or imagined) anal experience as possible. Do you crave penetration? Slow or fast? Do you envision a toy, finger, or penis moving in and out, side to side, or simply holding still? What kind of lube would you like? What sort of toys would you use?

Now, be even *more* specific and direct. What combinations and sequences of anal play work for you? For example, you might say, "Penis first, then butt plug, followed by more penis, and then dildo play internally." Or, "Oral sex on clitoris and vulva and then anus, followed by a finger on the outside of the anus with a dildo in the vagina." Alternatively, "Once something goes inside my butt, make sure to stimulate my clitoris."

Let's assume that you've had an awesome conversation about anal sex today, or last week, and both of you were enthusiastically on the same page. Now, here you are in the moment, all hot and heavy and ready to go. The last thing you want is to do something that freaks your partner out, and that can happen more often than you'd think, even if you've just had a positive discussion about anal sex. Why? Well, maybe your partner thought it would happen only in the distant future or after she or he played with your ass first. Or maybe your partner thought the anal-play discussion was only hypothetical and is thinking, "I've got no problem with the idea of butt play—in theory." Therefore, while it may seem redundant to ask again in the heat of the moment, it's important to say, "Is it okay to put my finger [or cock or toy] inside now?" Asking for consent at this point can help your partner feel respected, no matter how many times you've already done whatever you're doing. And, of course, it never hurts to use sexy language like, "Your butt looks so delicious right now. I hope you'll let me put my finger in so I can make you feel even hotter." Naturally, you'll hope that the answer is yes, but the fact is, there's a chance you'll get a no, even if you've discussed anal play already. Maybe your partner ate something spicy for lunch; maybe he's had irregular BMs that day; perhaps she hasn't had a chance to clean herself first; or maybe he just doesn't feel like it at the moment. All of those reasons are perfectly valid, and they're not a reflection on you. But sometimes we resist asking because we're afraid of a negative response that could make us feel rejected or stupid. Here's a way to handle that. Mike Domitrz, founder of *The Date Safe Project* (www.datesafeproject.org), suggests responding with, "Thanks for being honest with me. I would hate to do something that makes you uncomfortable." That way, embarrassment is kept to a minimum, and you can move on while feeling good about yourself and about your partner's no. Follow up that statement with a proactive question, such as, "What else can I do to make you feel awesome?"

Keep in mind that consent is not always as straightforward as a yes-or-no response. Ever been on the receiving end of a hug you felt obliged to accept from a family member or friend? Or, on a date, perhaps someone's asked, "Can I kiss you?" and you were so taken aback that you muttered a vague, "Umm . . . I guess so." If these situations sound familiar to you, you know from experience that consent can be more than a little tricky. According to Domitrz, one way to ensure enthusiastic consent is to put the ball in your partner's court. Instead of saying, "Can I put my penis inside you now?" ask your partner to take charge of the timing, and say, "Let me know when you want me to put my penis inside your sexy butt." Or say, "Tell me when you're hot enough and want me to move my tongue to your sweet rosebud." Even more generally, you might say, "Tell me when you're up for exploring anal play." Giving your partner the opportunity to really reflect and respond when he or she is ready, whether that's now or later, takes the pressure off both of you in the moment. Gaining your partner's active consent in these ways will help you feel confident that she or he is definitely excited for anal play.

FROM OUR SURVEY

" *Be open to experimenting, be open to being playful, and be open to the kind of communication that works best for your partner. Some people are super-chatty and some are not, and things are very seldom 'perfect' at first.* "

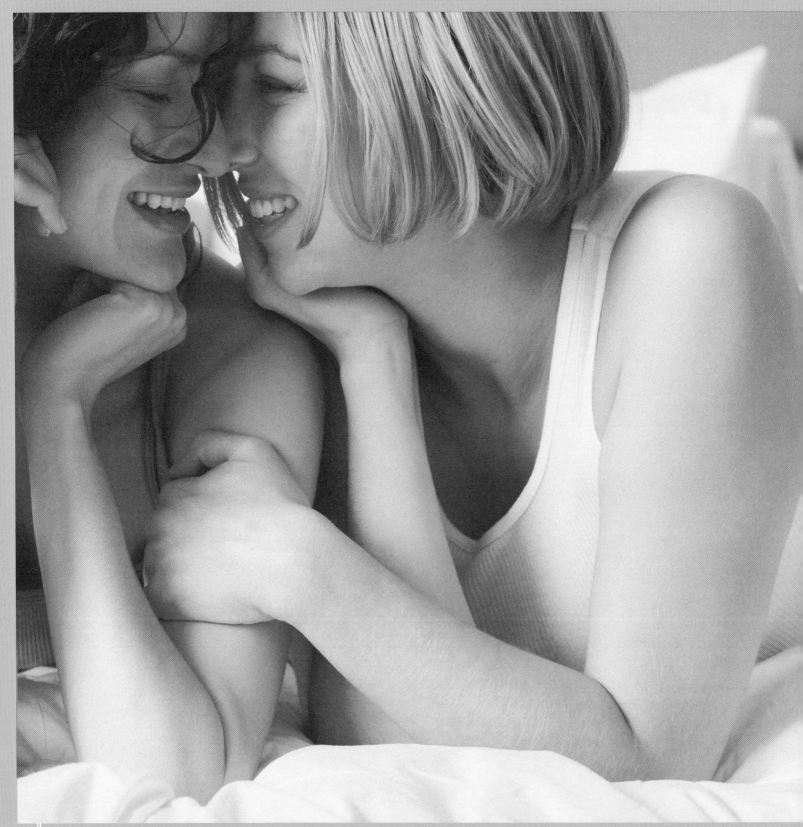

GREAT COMMUNICATION DURING ANAL SEX

Part of the beauty of anal play is that you usually can't see what your partner is doing—but wow, it feels amazing! So, when you're receiving anal pleasure, ask your partner to describe what she or he is doing so that you can ask for it again. You might even want to come up with names for different techniques. Say, "That feels amazing, hon. Tell me what you're doing so I can bribe you to do it again next time!"

By the same token, when you're on the giving end, describe what you're doing out loud, and do it seductively. Use your own words, of course, but you might say something along the lines of, "Your ass looks so hot. My fingers feel the pulsing of your sweet butt. It feels so good inside. I'm rotating my fingers around so I can feel every inch of you." You don't have to talk the whole time, but occasional comments like this help your partner visualize as well as feel what you're doing.

As a giver, nothing is sexier than hearing your partner tell you how great your magic touch makes her or him feel—but all givers need a little direction. And it's actually very easy to give your partner that direction while making her feel skilled and appreciated. Most important, be as specific as possible. When you're receiving pleasure, tell your partner exactly what works and what you want her or him to do differently. Many of us hold back on giving feedback in the moment for fear of "ruining" the whole encounter or insulting our partners. (And many of us even forget to tell our partners what feels good, assuming that it's perfectly obvious.) Instead, try combining the "positive" and "negative" feedback explicitly. Your partner will probably be very receptive to it. Here's how. . . .

Tell your partner something you like about what she or he is doing, followed by something you'd like her or him to do differently. Be specific (there's that phrase again!) about the speed, pressure, depth, rhythm, technique, angle, or level of lubrication. For example, you might say, "I love that level of speed, but could you go a little more gently?" Or, "There's enough lube, but please angle the toy [or finger or penis] toward my belly button." You can also say, "The pressure is great, but it feels a little too deep," or "I love your fingers on the outside, but I think I'd like it even better if you kept up the same technique and rhythm for a bit." The advantage of this strategy is twofold. First, you're giving your partner a positive response, which helps boost his or her confidence. Second, he or she will know what needs to be changed and what doesn't—and that means that his or her technique will improve the next time.

It's important to communicate your response to your partner, but it's equally important not to give up if the experience isn't perfect the first time. Sometimes, what happens is this: You ask your partner for a gentler pressure—say, a 3 on a scale of 1–10. Your partner was applying pressure at a level 8 and reduces the pressure to a 6 in response to your feedback—but that's not what you asked for. Lots of people get frustrated at this point and assume that their partners aren't really listening or that asking again isn't worth it. The result? You end up enduring less-than-awesome sex, which isn't fulfilling for you and wouldn't be fulfilling for your partner, if he or she knew how you felt. So don't give up right away. If you're in a situation like this, recognize that your partner *is* trying—she or he reduced the pressure from an 8 to a 6—and take this as evidence that your partner just needs a little more direction and clarification. You can use a 1–10 scale to help your partner understand the gradations in pressure. You might say, "You were at an 8 and reduced the pressure to a 6—but would you please go even more gently and drop it to a 3?" Or you can acknowledge your partner's effort and reframe your request in another way: "That *is* gentler. Can you do it even *more* gently, please?" Keep giving positive directions until you get exactly what you want.

The silent partner

You might be in a relationship in which your partner is unable to give you any feedback other than "It's fine"—despite the fact that you encourage him or her to speak up and tell you what he or she likes. Nonspecific comments like "It's fine" are hard to translate; they can mean anything from "Keep going," or "That's tolerable," to "I can just about stand it." If you want to coax more feedback from a silent partner, consider the possibility that your partner may not feel that it's safe to give more specific responses. So avoid asking questions like "Do you like this?" or "Is that okay?" Your partner might feel that it's difficult to answer such queries, because they seem to demand a yes-or-no response and may carry value judgments along with them. Instead, give your partner options. Ask, "Do you want it faster or slower?" or "Do you prefer it like this, or like that?" This will make it easier for your partner to respond because no matter which response he or she gives, his or her answer won't imply that one felt *bad*; one just didn't feel as good as the other one. Alternatively, try asking your partner to rate a bunch of different but similar things on a scale from 1 to 10. For example, when touching externally on the rosebud, ask for a numbered rating on each technique: small circular movements, larger circles, up-and-down strokes, windshield-wiper movement, or scissoring fingers. That way, you'll be more able to differentiate between them and to repeat a "fine" that rates a 9 rather than a "fine" that rates a 3.

Sexy it up

If telling your partner "I want to put a dildo up your butt" sounds boring, never fear: you can easily sexy up your language without sounding too cheesy or unnatural. Play fast and loose with adjectives and adverbs. A butt can become a sexy, hot, awesome, cute, handsome, beautiful, pretty, sweet, irresistible, dirty, horny, and/or hungry butt, depending on the mood you're looking to set and the words that turn you both on. Likewise, you can slowly, eagerly, gently, forcefully, delicately, voraciously, excitedly, or lovingly put something inside your partner's tender butt.

Brainstorm with your partner to decide on the names or nicknames you like to use for various body parts, such as vulva, vagina/innie, penis/outie, or butt. Agree on terms that neither of you find offensive (unless, of course, that's the effect you're both going for!) and that turn you on. Once you've got the vocabulary, you're well on your way to making anal play even hotter. You might say, "I love thrusting my big cock in your hot ass," or "I want to feel those skilled fingers inside me," or "Tell me when your hungry butt is ready for me." While you might not want to use these exact phrases, a little brainstorming and creativity is all it takes to get comfortable with dirty talk that can enhance the whole experience for both of you. If you start with just one new adjective and use words that feel genuine, you'll feel less awkward. And, as with most things, the more you practice, the easier it becomes.

FROM OUR SURVEY

Describe what you're going to do as you begin your seduction, maybe while you're stroking and massaging the ass and anal area. This can give your partner a chance to consent—or not—to your plan! Find a way to talk about it afterward. What worked? What was tricky? How could things have been better? Next time, apply what you've learned. Not sure if someone wants anal play? Offer it, and then ask your partner to beg you when she or he is ready!

" *I once went ahead without enough communication, mixed with nerves, resulting in an embarrassing sexual encounter where I prematurely inserted a butt plug into the ass of a beginner anal player, without warming the plug or my partner enough beforehand. I learned the hard way!* "

DEBRIEF

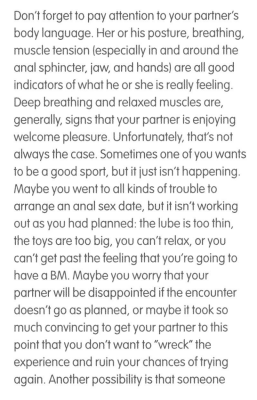

BODY LANGUAGE

Don't forget to pay attention to your partner's body language. Her or his posture, breathing, muscle tension (especially in and around the anal sphincter, jaw, and hands) are all good indicators of what he or she is really feeling. Deep breathing and relaxed muscles are, generally, signs that your partner is enjoying welcome pleasure. Unfortunately, that's not always the case. Sometimes one of you wants to be a good sport, but it just isn't happening. Maybe you went to all kinds of trouble to arrange an anal sex date, but it isn't working out as you had planned: the lube is too thin, the toys are too big, you can't relax, or you can't get past the feeling that you're going to have a BM. Maybe you worry that your partner will be disappointed if the encounter doesn't go as planned, or maybe it took so much convincing to get your partner to this point that you don't want to "wreck" the experience and ruin your chances of trying again. Another possibility is that someone

who is usually the "penetrator" might find that being penetrated as a bottom or being more vulnerable is more emotionally challenging than he or she expected. The reality is, sex doesn't always work out the way you planned it. Sometimes it's better; other times, it's disappointing. That's where body language comes in. Reading your partner's body language can help you determine whether a "Yes, keep going" is an enthusiastic request to move forward or whether it's masking a desire to stop. Reassure your partner (and yourself) that you can stop anytime, that there's no shame in discovering and naming a boundary, and that you'd rather shift gears than continue to do something that neither one of you enjoys. And there's a major plus side to all this: As you process the experience together afterward, you might discover new things about yourself and each other—and you might even reach a deeper level of intimacy than you'd thought possible.

On a regular basis, and every time you try something new, check in on how the sex was. Use the Three Oranges and a Lemon prompt (page 95) to talk about what worked and didn't work. Reassure your partner about what you love about him or her, regardless of how the session ended. It makes great post-sex cuddle talk and can ensure that you don't forget all of the aspects that worked really well and what you learned to fix or adjust for next time. That said, we tend to be very emotionally open and vulnerable after sex, so if there was something that really went wrong, sometimes it helps to wait 24 hours to talk about it. Unless you need to clear the air immediately, having hard discussions right after sex can be more emotional. If it can wait, give it some time for reflection, find the right words, and let it all sink in. Reid's conversation formula on page 96 is a great way to plan out and initiate that hard conversation. Good communication solidifies a relationship and opens the door for a more robust sex life. Now that you've discussed your likes and dislikes with your partner and resolved any issues, you can safely experiment with new tricks and techniques. Chapter 7 will help you with that. Read on to learn about some exciting positions and the promise of spectacular anal sex.

Chapter 7

POSITIONS:
INTERCOURSE, ORAL, AND FINGERS/TOYS

Comfortable and creative positioning can make the difference between good sex and great sex. It can also make the difference between feeling relaxed afterward and the need for a remedial back massage instead. As always, it is important to check in with your body during any kind of activity. It is especially important to be aware of your body when having sex. Any kind of sexual arousal increases our pain tolerance, such that we can be harming our bodies without even noticing until the endorphins wear off. Although some might argue that it is worth it, if physical pain can be avoided, then it totally begs consideration.

As a giver of pleasure, or top, your back is the most likely body part to cause problems. Hunching over a partner for any extended length of time or attempting new, wild positions makes many people's backs ache. So it is important to try to position yourself so that you are well-supported—whether lying on your back, side, or front; standing; or sitting up straight.

Beds are really convenient places to have sex; they can't be beat for a comfy mattress and options for positioning. Props can help make this perfect spot even more ideal. Pillows or shapes like the Liberator Wedge (which doesn't squish down like pillows do) can be a big help for either partner. Using one of these supports as a top can get you into a more effective position particularly for a marathon sex session. Or they can be used to prop up your receiver, or bottom, so that you're both comfortable while still having access to all of the important erogenous zones in his or her genitals and butt.

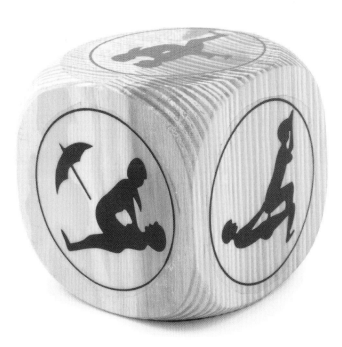

FROM OUR SURVEY

At a play party in just the last few weeks, I was finally able to find a heteroflexible fellow with a lovely thick, curved cock that was able to fuck me while I was recumbent on the edge of a massage table while I bore down on his in-strokes to help him hit all of the sweet spots.

Another comfortable strategy is using the side of the bed for positioning, with the bottom lying close to the edge and the top standing beside it, depending on your height and whether you have a low-lying futon or a tall bed that almost requires a ladder for access. Of course, a kitchen/bathroom counter, table, trunk of a car, or even a rock (for nature lovers) also work well (just add some soft padding!). Massage tables in particular are an overlooked yet fabulous sex accessory, offering padding for the receiver and comfort for the giver. When giving focused attention on a partner, being able to stand up and lean without straining is way more comfortable than trying to prop yourself up on your elbows, or sitting next to a partner. The good news is that folding massage tables are now affordable and easy to find. Even a secondhand one used by a retired massage therapist can be worth its weight in gold. Alternatively, a sex sling is an awesome bedroom accessory for those who really want their bedroom (or sex room) to be a lair of pleasure. A good sling with four points of anchoring to the ceiling can go up in minutes once the connections are safely positioned above. Some folks leave their slings up permanently if they have the space and don't have to worry about parents, kids, or housemates asking questions. Otherwise, taking it down is just as fast and leaves only eyebolts as evidence (which make nice places for hanging plants!).

Also, remember that the bottom's prostate, perineal sponge, and/or G-spot (referred to as PPG from here forward for brevity!) are stimulated through the front wall of the rectum. This means the best way to angle a toy or penis is to insert it as though you were trying to hit the belly button through the rectum. Aiming toward the front of the body at the right depth can be the most exquisite sensation (disproving the "bigger is always better" theory). Sometimes a smaller toy or penis with the correct angle can rival any large option, which can be overwhelming or too large to be pleasurable.

Another consideration to remember is that the closer the receiver's knees are to his or her chest, the straighter the rectum, and so the easier it is to welcome a toy or penis into the butt pleasurably. Positions like these are generally preferable for all kinds of folks, but especially beginners.

POSITIONS FOR INTERCOURSE

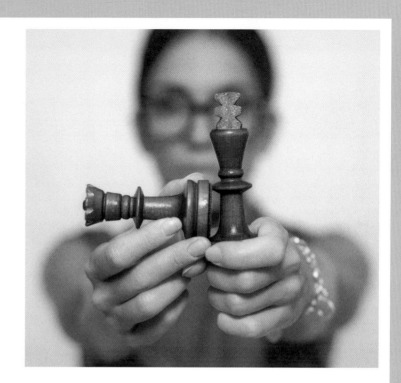

People who love intercourse *really love* intercourse. It is the most common sex act of all, whether it be anal or vaginal penetration. And folks are always looking for ways to spice it up with some variety, intimacy, and intensity. In this section are some recommended positions that can transform your anal sex experience. A very simple accessory can also help: the chest harness. Made in different styles, this accoutrement fits over the chest, around the breasts or covering the nipples. Not only does it look sexy, but it also enables the other partner to grab on to it for a more intense ride. The harness can be worn by either the top or bottom and can be used as a tool for dominance or just for practicality. For example, holding on to the harness can make it easier to thrust forcefully thanks to having something to grab (other than hair). It can also be used for non-intercourse activities, but this sex accessory really shines during penetration.

There are four main positions for intercourse, with infinite variations: missionary/bottom underneath, bottom on top, doggy/from behind, and standing/facing each other.

FROM OUR SURVEY

For butt play, squatting makes all sorts of things possible.

Missionary/bottom underneath

If thinking about missionaries getting it on while you have sex is not your fantasy, then "bottom underneath" is an alternative name for this popular position. The bottom lies on his or her back, and the top straddles over the bottom. If either wears a chest harness, the other can grab on to it for additional effect.

Advantages: This position offers good eye contact. The bottom is relaxed, making it easier to orgasm. Depending on the top's position, it may allow for penis or clitoral stimulation at the same time.

Disadvantages: The bottom cannot control the angle, depth, or speed of penetration. The top is often unable to sustain long sessions. Little physical touch is possible on the rest of the body.

VARIATIONS

1. The Pilates: The bottom rolls back, putting the weight on his or her shoulders and getting the butt in the air to make it easier to enter the correct hole (if there are two) and to angle better toward the PPG. The bottom's legs pull against the chest, go up in the air, or rest on the top's shoulders. This requires the top to sit back on his or her heels for the optimum angle for reaching the PPG.

2. The Ramp: A ramp under the butt means that the bottom can feel the benefits of the Pilates above but can relax rather than having an abdominal workout at the same time, thus making it easier to orgasm. It also takes some of the strain off the top to hold the up the bottom and allows easier clitoral or penis stimulation.

FROM OUR SURVEY

I like to lie on my back, faceup, so that we can see each other's facial expressions for intercourse. I prefer this for its intimacy and emotional pleasure.

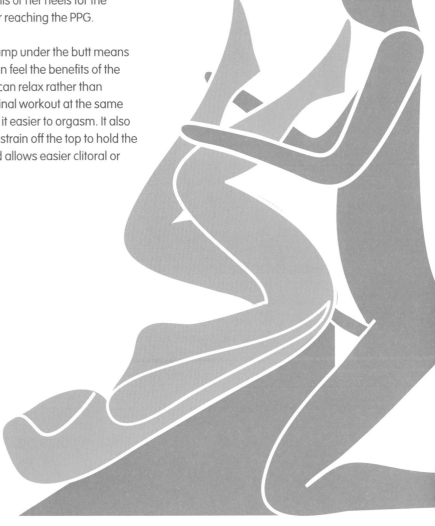

The Ramp

3. The Sandwich: The top faces and lies completely on top of the bottom, such that the full body contact and partner's weight feels intimate. This position is most effective and easiest to sustain if the bottom wraps his or her legs around the top's back. It can be a little tricky to maneuver, so you might have to get to this position via regular missionary. It is best for slower and shallower thrusting with more grinding against penises and clits, but there's not much room for other toys unless they are attached to the penis or dildo.

4. Thigh Harness: Lots more physical intimacy and full body touching are possible if you add a thigh harness, and thrusting is easier on the top, who can thus push harder and last longer. Each partner may even be able to wear his or her own thigh harness and penetrate each other at the same time! It's an alternative variation of double penetration!

5. The Sling: In a sling, the bottom can relax fully with his or her full body, including legs, supported and positioned so that the butt is at the optimum height and angle for the top's height. The top stands, holding two of the ropes or chains anchored above, and barely has to work in order to thrust because the sling swings back and forth in rhythm. This is an ideal configuration for the couple who like long, marathon anal sex sessions or who have bad backs. You can do slow, fast, deep, or shallow thrusting and additional stimulation on the penis, clit, vagina, and/or testicles. It all adjusts effortlessly for everyone's satisfaction.

FROM OUR SURVEY

We started our play in missionary, and that was good at first. After a little while, it felt awkward and exposing to me to be in that position for any length of time. I flipped over onto my tummy and squeezed my thighs tightly. I found lying on my stomach much more enjoyable and I was able to relax and receive much easier that way.

> *My go-to position is for me to be on top of my partner, cowgirl style. It allows me to have control, and that means I control how fast insertion happens and where the cock goes inside of me. It is the safest bet to prevent discomfort. However, I also like being fucked missionary though it's more likely to be uncomfortable, because in the proper circumstances, it can make penetration and withdrawal go more smoothly and it puts the power in my partner's hands.* "

Bottom on top

The top lies on his or her back, and the bottom climbs onto the top partner's penis or dildo. When the top wears a chest harness, the bottom can grab on to the harness for extra leverage.

Advantages: This position is fabulous for the bottom to take control of the timing, depth, and speed of penetration. It is also a great position for additional stimulation of the bottom's genitals and/or nipples/breasts/chest.

Disadvantages: It can be hard for the bottom to hold the position for a long time.

VARIATIONS

1. The Squat: The bottom squats, with feet on the ground (rather than kneeling). PPG pleasure is maximized when the bottom leans back, hands resting on the top's bent knees or on the bed/ground between the top's feet. It is hard, though, for many folks to orgasm when their thighs are on fire and shaking in an attempt to keep thrusting. To prevent or alleviate the bottom's thigh burn, this partner remains in one place, and the top does the thrusting or helps lift the other partner up and down with his or her hands.

2. The Reverse: The bottom is still on top but now faces the top's feet instead of his or her head. The top has a great view of the bottom's butt and the thrusting action and can massage around the anus with his or her fingers at the same time for added pleasure. The bottom either kneels or squats. This is also a great position for the bottom to play with the top's genitals and/or anus using hands or toys.

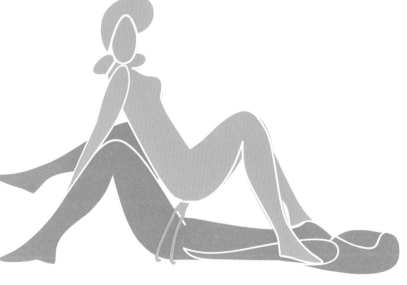

The Squat leaning backwards

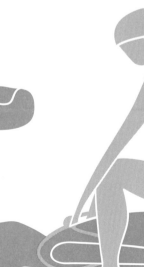

The Squat with chest harness

3. The Open-Faced Sandwich: The bottom faces the top's feet and then lies back so that he or she is fully lying down with his or her back against his or her partner's front. In this position, the knees are usually bent and the feet are flat on the ground. It's a very intimate position, with lots of options for touching and kissing the receiving partner. But it's a little challenging for fast, deep thrusting.

4. Thigh Harness: The bottom sits on the top's thigh while the latter either lies on his or her back with knees up or down, or sits down. Either partner can take an active role in the thrusting movement.

FROM OUR SURVEY

" I like to do it on top of and laying horizontally over my partner, who is also horizontal on his back, and lifting myself up and down over his body, with his penis inserted in my ass. Tricky but very hot. "

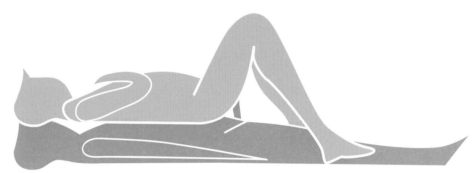

The Open-Faced Sandwich

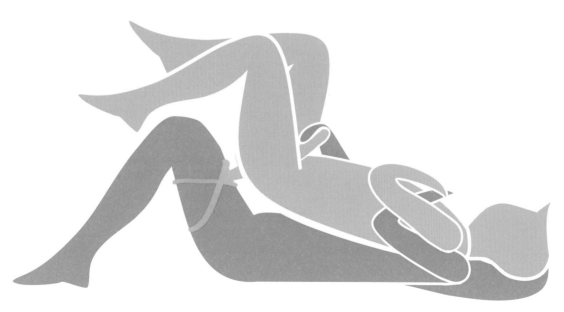

Thigh Harness

From behind: Classic "doggy-style"

The bottom gets on all fours, like a dog, and the top kneels behind.

Advantages: Some folks actually love the "animalistic" or taboo nature of this position (see "Disadvantages" for another take on this). The receiving partner can control the timing, depth, and speed of penetration at the beginning or all the way through, if desired. This position is generally good for additional clit/vagina/penis/testicle stimulation at the same time. When the bottom wears a chest harness, the top has something fun to grab hold of to add intensity. Doggy-style is excellent for PPG stimulation—as long as the top is taller than the bottom. If not, then the top has to either stand and squat (hard on the thighs), or the bottom needs to spread his or her legs or lean forward or back to lower the butt so that the top can enter from above, aiming down toward the bottom's belly button from inside.

Disadvantages: The temptation in this position is for the top to thrust quickly and deeply, which may not be pleasurable or desirable to the bottom. It requires some self-control on the part of the top (which can be distracting) to not get lost in the throes of passion and deep thrusting (which the bottom may or may not like). Some feel disconnected from their partner in this position because they can't see each other. Doing it in front of a full-length mirror brings back some of that connection and eroticism, as you can look at each other (and the two of you together!).

VARIATIONS

1. The Plank: The bottom lies on his or her stomach, with a pillow under the pelvis, raising his or her butt slightly in the air and keeping the back comfortable. The beauty of this position is that the depth of penetration is shallower because the bottom's butt cheeks are in the way, and the angle is such that the top aims specifically toward the front wall of the rectum, making it pretty hard not to hit the PPG. When penetrated by a penis, the bottom can squeeze his or her legs together around the penis for added stimulation of the shaft by the thighs. The top holds him- or herself up in a position similar to the strength exercise called the plank, which makes it a good workout but a position in which it's hard to last long. The bottom can lie on a toy to grind into, but there's not much room for other added pleasure.

FROM OUR SURVEY

When I am fucking someone, I like to have them in the most relaxed position possible for them—and that's different for everyone. One of my favorites is to have someone lying on their side, almost in a fetal position, with their ass sticking out. It's easy to relax like that, and I like pulling their ass apart to look at it. You can also fuck someone in a few different ways when they are lying like that: curled up behind them, which can be more tender, or kneeling above them, which can be a more aggressive fuck.

2. Squat Dog: Once in the doggy-style position, the top sits back on his or her heels, and the bottom leans back to squat on top of his or her partner, placing his or her hands on the ground/bed or on the headboard to brace him- or herself and make it easier to be more active.

3. Spoon Dog: Spooning is popular for the full-body touch that a couple can experience together as well as for putting hands on each other's bodies. It also is a great way to penetrate from behind, incorporating more body intimacy than with traditional doggy-style. It is a little harder to thrust quickly, which may not be preferable anyhow.

4. Thigh Dog: Similar to Spoon Dog, the top spoons the bottom from behind and uses a thigh harness that thrusts powerfully and easily. There are lots of full-body touching and kissing options in this position.

FROM OUR SURVEY

For anal sex, I find I often prefer any position coming in from behind, whether it's standing, doggy, or lying on the bed. It's comfortable, and there's a ton of body contact. People often counter that you don't get as much eye contact, which I guess is true, but I find I get enough eye contact most of the rest of the time. Fucking time is fucking time.

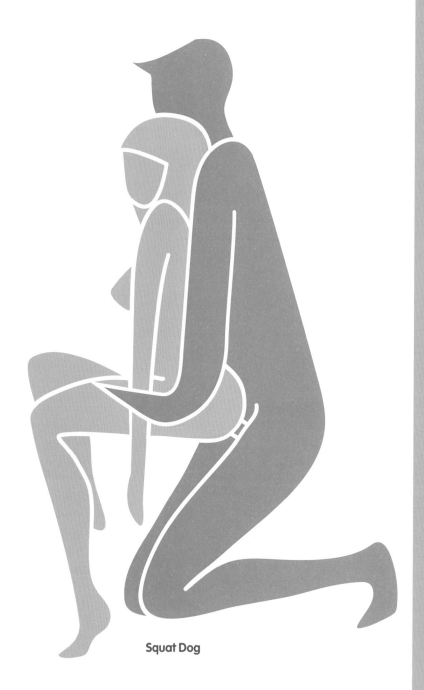

Squat Dog

Standing/facing each other

This position is a little more gymnastic, but fun. It can work well in the shower, in a stairwell, against a wall, or in midair for those who are really strong! Slings like the Sportsheets Door Jam Sex Sling alleviate some of the weight of the bottom to make it easier for the top to hold him or her up.

Advantages: Standing sex feels like superhero sex Olympics, which is fun. There's great eye contact and full-body alignment, plus options for kissing.

Disadvantages: This position is easiest when the bottom is a few inches taller than the top in order to make it work without the bottom

having to be picked up. It is really tiring for both partners and may even be impossible for many tops (especially to hold up their partners). Most of the top's energy goes into squatting to get underneath the bottom, or into not falling or dropping his or her partner if he or she picks up the bottom, so there's not much energy left for thrusting. This position is not effective for PPG angling.

VARIATIONS

1. The *W*: Facing each other with knees bent, use a double-ended dildo, each side in someone's butt. The best dildo for this purpose is actually not straight, but a mustache-shaped one made by Fun Factory. As each partner thrusts, the dildo bends in the middle, bumping up against the perineum and/or clitoris of each partner.

2. Yab/Yum: This classic tantric position is designed to line up the spiritual/sexual energy centers between partners. Facing each other but not standing, the top sits with his or her legs crossed while the bottom sits on the top's lap, legs wrapped around his or her back. If the bottom is slightly shorter than the top, then the heart, mouth, and other energy centers are connected at the same time as penetration, creating deeper intimacy. In a position that makes it a little hard to thrust, the movement here is less pronounced and sometimes even more circular or grinding.

For additional variations with descriptions and images of anal intercourse positions, see Tristan Taormino's *The Anal Sex Position Guide.*

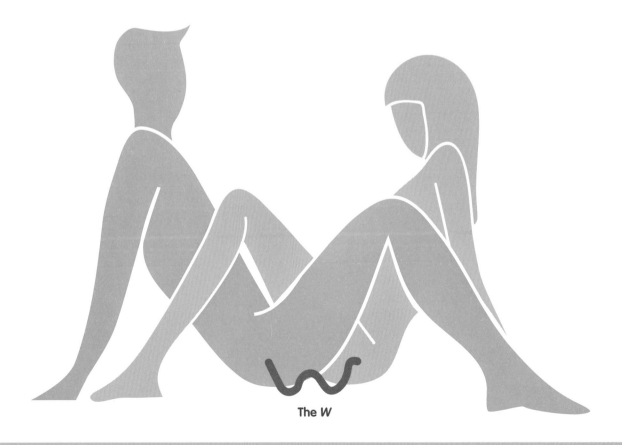

The *W*

FINGER/ TOY PLAY

FROM OUR SURVEY

" *I don't have a favorite position. If it's in me, I like it. I like both hand and toy play.* "

Being comfortable while using fingers and toys is equally important to positioning during intercourse. Sometimes we don't want to break the rhythm when our partner is close to climax. Starting off comfortably means that changing positions is less likely to need to happen at a disruptive time.

Taking turns

When the bottom is lying on his or her back, a super-comfortable position for the top is to sit between the partner's knees, the top's knees bent and over his or her partner's. A pillow (covered with a towel) under the bottom's butt gives a better view and access to the pleasure spots in and around the butt. The bottom can also lift his or her legs in the air and rest them on the chest or on the partner's shoulders for easier penetration and better PPG play. This presents lots of options for either partner to add hands or toys to the bottom's other erogenous zones. There is tons of eye contact in this position, which enables the giver to read the partner's reactions to the sensations better and build intimacy.

VARIATIONS

1. Doggy: The bottom is on all fours, as in doggy-style, and the top sits between the bottom's feet or beside one knee. The top can lean against the bottom and use his or her other hand to stimulate lots of other areas on the bottom's body.

Taking Turns

2. Flat Doggy: Like in the Plank, Flat Doggy has the bottom lie flat on the bed or table with a pillow under the pelvis, while the top sits between or beside the bottom's legs or stands next to the massage table or bed. This position is good for folks who also like to grind their clits/cocks into a vibrator or the bed.

3. Fetal Position: The bottom is on his or her side in the fetal position, and the top is standing (if using a massage table) or lying behind him or her, either pointing the same way or pointing toward the feet. This position enables some full-body contact during anal play.

4. Sixty-Nine: Of course oral can be added, but this version of Sixty-Nine involves both partners being stimulated on the anus, vagina, penis, and/or testicles at the same time with fingers and/or toys. It can be tricky for both partners to see what they are doing to each other, especially if they are both doing anal play; however, the taller partner often has the visual advantage.

5. Sling: The bottom literally hangs out, comfortably lying back in the sling, while the penetrating partner sits relaxed on a chair with excellent access to the butt and other erogenous zones. This is a great position for the long haul.

FROM OUR SURVEY

" *I love it in a sling, legs spread and up in the air.* "

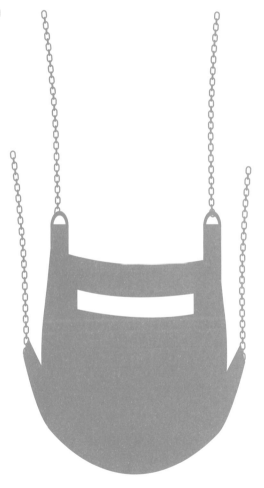

Sling

ORAL POSITIONS

Oral is always a fabulous combination with butt play: oral on the anus and/or oral on the genitals while toys and fingers roam the anal and rectal regions is a particular delight.

1. Missionary/Bottom on the Bottom: Prop up the bottom on pillows to ease the pressure on the top's neck and provide better access to the butt. The bottom can bring his or her knees to the chest to make it easier on everyone. If the bottom is in the sling or at the edge of the bed with legs over the top's shoulders, the top can sit in a chair for maximum comfort and endurance.

2. Brunch: The bottom straddles—basically sits on—the top's face. The bottom needs to be mindful to not put all of his or her weight on the top, which can lead to straining the partner's neck or suffocating him or her! If facing the top's head, the bottom can lean partway or even all the way back to get his or her anus in the right spot. When the bottom lies all the way back, such that the back of the bottom's head is resting on the top's genitals, it is super comfortable for both. If straddling the opposite way—facing the top's feet instead—the bottom can lean comfortably forward onto his or her hands. In any of these options, either partner can use his or her hands for added stimulation of either or both partner's nipples/breasts, other genitals, and other parts of the body.

3. Sixty-Nine: This position involves oral and fingers and toys on all parties at the same time. Allow yourself time-outs to simply receive pleasure, rather than feeling like you need to be active the whole time. It can be easier to orgasm, for example, when taking a break for a few minutes. Many have a hard time concentrating on giving and receiving at the same time and need to focus on only one when it gets intense. Do this position on top of each other or side by side.

4. A Dog's Breakfast: For this doggy-style play, the bottom is on all fours, butt in the air. The giver kneels for a great view of the anus and excellent access around the front to all the other delicacies that await on the other side. The bottom can grind him- or herself backward into the giver's face to control the pressure and tongue variations. Either partner can use his or her hands or toys on the bottom's genitals.

5. Spoon-Fed: One partner lies in a fetal position on his or her side while the other lies just behind, pointing the same way or the opposite way. This position offers great access to all of the erogenous zones, especially if the receiving partner puts one knee toward his or her chest, opening up the butt cheeks and pelvis to opportunities for pleasure.

If any position becomes uncomfortable or boring, switch it up. Sometimes you just need to change the angle or add a prop. There are no rules about staying in place once you start. Variety is the spice of life, and switching up positions and angles keeps everyone interested and excited. Feel free to let your partner know: "I am not done with you yet. I need to change position so that I can comfortably give you all the pleasure you can handle."

Chapter 8
TOYS, LUBES, AND CONDOMS:
MAXIMIZING SAFETY AND PLEASURE

Toys are great anal-play accessories. In fact, when it comes to anal, using toys is practically a necessity. It can be hard to stimulate your butt in all the ways you'd like to when you're just working with your hands—unless you're a human pretzel, that is! Sharing your toys with your partner is fun and exciting, and if you're flying solo, toys make it so much easier to play.

If you're brand-new to anal pleasure, use your fingers to explore your butt before you move on to a toy. Those sensitive nerves in your fingers can really help you get a sense of your body's geography. And your digits are far more versatile in terms of angle and flexibility than any toy could ever be. Once you know your anus and rectum inside and out—literally!—you're ready to go toy shopping.

That's where this chapter comes in. It'll help you figure out which toys you'd like to take with you on your anal adventures and will give you a crash course in using condoms and other safer-sex supplies that make for healthy anal play. It'll show you why all lubes aren't created equal—and lots more. Let's start with a rundown of what most sex toys are made of.

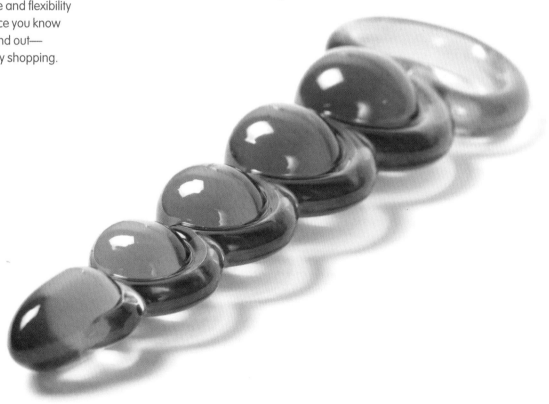

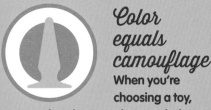

Color equals camouflage

When you're choosing a toy, remember that toys that are dark in color tend to camouflage bits of poop that might linger on them after use—and that can be a good thing. But it does mean it's less obvious when they're dirty. (Plus, dirt can accumulate in the crevices of some toys.) Think about using black condoms over your toys: it's a simple way to minimize visible mess and make cleanup quick and easy.

FROM OUR SURVEY

" One challenge I have with toys is that my eyes are sometimes bigger than my ass. I'm not sure I have totally overcome this. Sometimes this is still true, but I realize that sometimes I am more relaxed and able to take bigger objects than at other times. "

CHOOSING MATERIALS

Because sex toys are an unregulated industry, you need to mind your health by being a savvy shopper. Watch out for the disclaimer "For novelty purposes only," which appears on the packaging for a lot of sex toys (especially the less-expensive ones). This means that the product is intended as a gag gift, so if you use it for sexual stimulation and end up with health problems as a result, the manufacturer won't be liable. This is an incredibly dishonest trick since, of course, it's obvious to everyone that such toys are in fact produced and marketed for sex play. So steer clear of toys that come with that disclaimer. Be sure to buy your toys from reputable companies, seek out retailers that take pride in giving their customers honest information (check out the resources section for suggestions), and use your toys safely. That's the best way to enjoy pleasurable, safe anal sex adventures.

Softer materials

One of the great things about soft toys is that they're flexible, which is especially important when it comes to butt play. And they make thrusting and deep penetration more comfortable. Soft toys are likely to be made of . . .

PVC, rubber, latex, or "jelly." Toys made from these materials have several major advantages. They're soft, flexible, and inexpensive. But they've got serious downsides, too. They don't last as long as other materials (like silicone, metal, or glass), they discolor easily, and they're porous, which means they're difficult to clean thoroughly— and that can lead to STIs or bacterial infections. And they can "interact" with each other, which means if they're stored together, they might "melt" each other and get ruined. Plus, lots of folks try to avoid latex, either due to allergies or to prevent a latex sensitivity from developing due to overexposure.

Soft toys have another grave disadvantage, too. Many contain phthalates, which are softening agents that have been linked to infertility, cancer, and birth defects in some studies. (In fact, in 2012, the United States Congress banned phthalates in toys for children due to these health concerns.) Phthalates are particularly worrisome because they don't bind to the material to which they're added, so they leach into whatever touches them. You'll probably know whether a toy contains phthalates thanks to its signature scent, which is intense and awfully headache-inducing. (If you've ever bought a cheap shower curtain, you'll know what I mean!) Happily, the sex toy industry has responded to consumer awareness, and many toys these days sport labels designating them "phthalate-free."

If you already have any PVC, rubber, latex, or jelly toys, always store them in separate bags and use a condom with them to lower health risks and to keep your toy completely clean. If you do need to wash your toy, use nonoily soap and water. These toys can be used with water- and silicone-based lubricants.

Elastomer, including TPE (thermoplastic elastomer) or TPR (thermoplastic rubber). These polymers are great alternatives to latex. They're made without the allergy-inducing proteins that latex contains, and they're phthalate-free, too. But they're still usually porous, so it's best to use a condom with them to keep them as clean as possible. Like PVC toys, they can be cleaned with nonoily soap and water and can be used with water- and silicone-based lubes.

CyberSkin/Ultraskin/UR3. A soft, phthalate-free material that's popular for its looks, this feels a lot like real skin. Watch out, though. This material is extremely porous and feels tacky after it's washed. To keep that tacky feeling at bay, toys made of these substances usually come with a powder to sprinkle on them post-washing. Some people aren't convinced that the powder is safe and use cornstarch instead. Use toys made from these materials with a condom, or clean them with nonoily soap and water. Remember that CyberSkin toys can only be used with water-based lubricants.

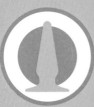

Should you share your toys?

Well, when it comes to sex toys—particularly toys used during anal sex—sharing is not necessarily caring. It's usually fine if you and your partner aren't concerned about STIs, but not when it comes to anal play. That's because toys can easily transmit bacteria (like E. coli) or parasites, not to mention STIs. Make this your mantra: one toy, one butt. If you still want to share, you can use fresh condoms on the toy for each partner. Or, if your toy is made from 100 percent silicone, metal, or glass and has no vibrating mechanism, you can sterilize it by boiling it. Here's how: wash your toy first, and then submerge it in a pot of boiling water for 3 minutes. Be sure to set the timer; many a forgotten toy has been boiled down into a mangled, unusable shape after the water in the pot evaporates! Once your toy's been boiled, it's ready to be shared with a new lover (or to be loaned to a friend).

Silicone. This is the premium material for soft sex toys. It's flexible, durable, hypoallergenic, and nonporous, and it can be sterilized by boiling in water for at least 3 minutes. It also conducts vibration easily, so it easily turns into a vibrating toy if you place your vibe against the base. Some come with a vibrator included! If you're into vigorous play, it's the ideal choice. Silicone produced by different manufacturers may be more or less soft. Adult toy manufacturer Vixen Creations (www.vixencreations.com) started a trend when it created dual-density silicone VixSkin, a material that has a firm core to help the toy keep its shape surrounded by a softer type of silicone that's super comfortable for play—and which feels a lot like a real penis. In general, silicone toys are on the expensive side, because the raw material is more costly, but most consumers feel that the quality and safety is worth the extra cash. Sex toys are an unregulated industry, though, which means that some toys labeled "silicone" may actually contain as little as 10 percent silicone. It's a sneaky way for the producer to cut manufacturing costs. Fortunately, trustworthy brands like LELO, Jimmyjane, Vibratex, Fun Factory, Standard Innovation (We-Vibe), JOPEN, Happy Valley/Fuze, Tantus, and Vixen all use the best-quality silicone in their toys.

Firmer materials

Toys that are rigid are awesome for pinpoint pleasure: they can really hit the spots that are most enjoyable. But they can be painful or even harmful when they poke the rectum, so use them with care. Firm toys are best for experienced anal aficionados who can distinguish between a different-but-pleasurable sensation and a different-and-harmful one. They're best for slow, subtle movements, not fast thrusting. And they also conduct vibration really well, so you can add variation to anal play by placing your vibe against the outside of the toy.

ABS plastic makes durable, affordable toys that conduct vibration really well. Many vibrators are made from this material. Some then add a thin outer layer of silicone for a slick, velvety texture. Clean toys made from ABS plastic—which is compatible with water- and silicone-based lubricants—with a noncreamy soap and water.

FROM OUR SURVEY

"*I didn't like using silicone dildos because they felt too hard—until I tried a VixSkin. It's soft in all the right places, but it's firm enough to get the job done!*"

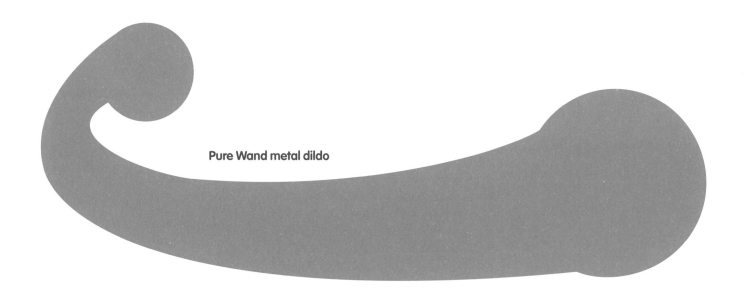

Pure Wand metal dildo

Metal toys are smooth, heavy, stylish, and indestructible—and that's what makes them so popular. They're nonporous and can easily be sterilized in boiling water for extra safety or for sharing with a partner. (If you do boil your metal toy to sterilize it, remember that metal retains heat for quite a while, so to avoid burning yourself, don't use it directly after boiling!) Use any water-, silicone-, or oil-based lube with metal toys, and clean them by washing them with a soap of your choice.

Glass, Pyrex, and acrylic—don't worry: glass toys are sturdier than they sound! A solid glass toy shouldn't break unless you drop it from several feet onto a hard floor. If that happens, here's what to do: run your hands over it (as if you were giving it a hand job) to feel for any nicks. If your hand doesn't feel any, then neither will your body, so it's safe to use. A glass toy won't break while you're using it inside your body unless you have Superman-style sphincter muscles. (If you can't break your toy in half with your hands,

neither can your sphincters.) Lots of glass toys are also lovely to look at. These objets d'art make fine coffee-table decorations. Glass is heavier and tends to look more attractive. Acrylic and Pyrex are less weighty, but are also durable and pretty. All of these materials are nonporous and can be used with any type of lubricant—and their smooth texture means a little lube goes a long way. Wash them with any soap of your choice.

Wood is a lightweight material that embodies elegance and pleasure. Wooden toys are tough and durable, and as long as they're coated with a body-safe lacquer to prevent splintering, they're ready to use immediately. They can be used with water-, oil-, or silicone-based lubricants and can be washed with any type of gentle soap.

FROM OUR SURVEY

I'm a huge fan of steel toys because they're super-smooth, easy to clean, last forever, and they look great. They can be used in sensation play with a little heat or cold, and they just slip right in without requiring a ton of lube. The Njoy Pure Wand is my favorite toy in my extensive toy collection.

TOY STYLES

Now that you're familiar with toy materials, you can decide which type of toy is right for you. It depends on the type of sensation you're looking for.

Anal beads. Lots of anal-play rookies choose anal beads as their first toy. Anal beads are a series of (usually silicone) beads designed to be inserted during arousal and pulled out at the point of orgasm to heighten pleasure. Strings of anal beads can be long or short, and the beads themselves may be smaller or larger, which produce different sensations. The feelings they create come from the way your anal sphincter muscles open and close over the balls. What is unique about these rippled toys is that they massage and stimulate the sphincters from both directions: on the way in and out. Most anal beads are very floppy, and you need to use both hands to insert them. That makes them less practical, because once they're out, you'll need both your hands to put them back in again—which means that both of your hands will get dirty. So unless you use disposable gloves or stop play to wash your hands, you're more likely to spread E. coli or hepatitis during the rest of the encounter. To make life a bit easier, try using a firm set of beads that can be deployed using one hand instead of two. Plus, with firm beads, you can achieve an in-and-out motion more easily. Just don't go too fast, as the variation in the width of the beads could tear the anus. On the upside, though, if you're after an intense session, you won't need to work as hard.

FROM OUR SURVEY

The Lust beads have fabulous vibration, very strong and smooth. The flexibility of the toy creates a lot of options: prostate stimulation, different angles, and different lengths. Stays in place so you can put it in and then do other things with your hands. Very versatile.

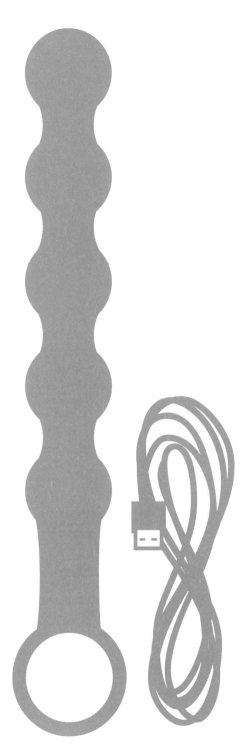

Lust L 4.5 anal beads with charging cord

Butt plugs. A butt plug is a toy that's designed to "plug" the anus. It stays in place after it's inserted. Butt plugs have a signature look. They're usually shaped like the ace in a deck of cards. They're likely to have a tapered tip that widens toward the middle and then slims down to a narrow neck before flaring out again at the base. A comfortable plug will have a long, thin base that nestles nicely between the butt cheeks, rather than a round base that pries the butt cheeks open. You need a long-enough neck so that the sphincters have enough room to rest in the neck of the toy. Toys with short necks or necks that aren't much narrower than the middle tend to be pushed out rather than held in place (sphincter muscles are hardwired to push things out). Some plugs with extra-long necks can also be used for shallow in-and-out thrusting, but generally, plugs are designed to be left in place. Here's why they're pleasurable: When a toy is inserted, the anal sphincters are left open rather than closed, and because of the heightened sensitivity in the area, even small movements of your legs or pelvis can make the toy shift slightly, gently adjusting the anal tissue surrounding the toy.

A plug also allows the sphincters to get used to being open and teaches them to relax around the width of the toy. That's why it's often used as a stepping-stone to inserting something wider. If you want to have anal intercourse, for example, try inserting progressively larger plugs, and leave each one in place for a few minutes with some genital play in between. That'll allow the sphincters to relax gradually around greater widths. (Note that this doesn't "stretch" the sphincter muscles, as the feeling is often incorrectly described; it simply relaxes them.) Then, after a toy is removed from the rectum, the anal sphincter won't close immediately. It takes about a minute to close fully. (Ever hopped into the shower to wash right after having a BM, and noticed that your anus is still open a little?) Progressively inserting another toy or penis of a slightly larger width is much easier to accomplish pleasurably than going from zero to sixty—that is, closed anus to penis width—in an instant. Regular butt players might be able to take a toy or penis that's 1–2 inches (2.5–5 cm) wide without much warmup and experience no pain, but they're a minority. And there's no shame in taking the time you need to gradually, painlessly open up to a pleasurable width.

Dildos. These long baton- or phallus-shaped toys are designed for penetration or thrusting, and many are made to be used in a harness. (Find out how to use a dildo with a harness on page 135.) Some are uniform in width, which is ideal if you're new to anal play, since they're easier to manage when it comes to faster movement. Dildos with variations in width, such as ridges or curvy waves, provide a more intense experience. They tire out the sphincters much faster and often require more frequent lube applications. Curved dildos are great for stimulating the G-spot or P-spot. Different folks have different aesthetic preferences for their toys. Some like their dildos to look like penises, while others prefer a less phallic association and go for toys that resemble a goddess, a dolphin—or nothing at all. Dildos with tapered heads make for easy entry. Those with pronounced heads are a little harder to get in, but once they're there, you can gently pull the bulb against the anal

opening for extra sensation before you pull all the way out. Pronounced heads also make thrusting more practical, as you don't need to worry about pulling all the way out by accident. (After all, if you're thrusting away like a sex superstar in the heat of the moment, having your partner inform you that you're actually humping the air by mistake might be more than a little embarrassing!) Also, unlike most butt plugs, most dildos need to be held in place; your sphincter muscles will push them out otherwise.

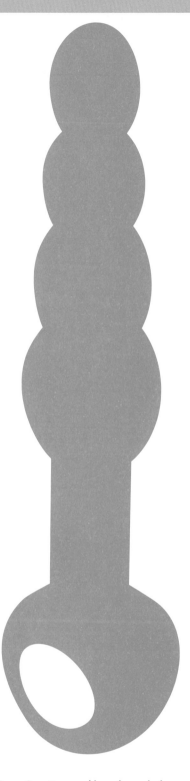

Fuze Quattro anal beads and plug

> **FROM OUR SURVEY**
>
> *❝ I used the Quattro in conjunction with a vibrator on my clit. This might be too intense for some people, but it really did the trick for me! The sensation was incredible, and despite not having tried anal sex for more than 5 years, I was able to comfortably receive 3 inches on the first try. ❞*

The curve of the Slow Drive was great for G-spot play, but it was also very easy and enjoyable to use for back-and-forth anal play, which surprised me. I think more practice with this toy could make me much more comfortable with actual penis insertion, which is a big deal for me.

A soft dildo used for thrusting is usually preferable to a firm one—but beware of those that are too soft. In general, the longer and thinner a dildo is, the less rigid it is, which means that it might buckle or "give" during penetration in the same way that a semi-erect penis would. The key is to strike a balance between hard and soft. You may need to buy a few dildos and experiment with them before you find your ideal toy.

Some dildos also come with a suction cup at the base. This way, the wall, the floor, or another firm, flat surface can be your partner. But you're the one who needs to do the thrusting!

Of course, when you're buying any toy for anal play, you need to make sure that your eyes aren't wider than your butt. That thick dildo may *look* sexy, but it might be too wide for you, especially if you're a beginner. So be realistic. There's no shame in starting small! It's better to stick to a comfortable size than to find yourself unable to enjoy the pleasure or to have to limit thrusting just to cope with the width of your new toy.

Vibrators. Made to stimulate sensitive spots like vaginas, butts, clits, anuses, or penises, vibrators typically have multiple settings for different degrees of intensity. Some people love the sensation, others don't; some folks use vibrators on some parts of the body, but not on others. Consider giving it a go against or inside your butt, even if you don't typically like vibration elsewhere. You might be pleasantly surprised!

There's just one thing that can compromise vibrator-induced anal pleasure: becoming numb to the sensations. Here's how that happens. When you find that special spot with your vibrator, it's so tempting to stay there. After all, if it feels good, why put it anywhere else? The thing is, though, that repetition can numb your senses. For instance, if a friend or partner rubs your arm in the same way for more than a minute, the amazing sensation you felt at first quickly fades into the background. Or if you walk out into a noisy street after chatting with a friend in a quiet café, you'll notice the contrast in environments at first, but your brain will soon adjust to the new level of background sound. Your body

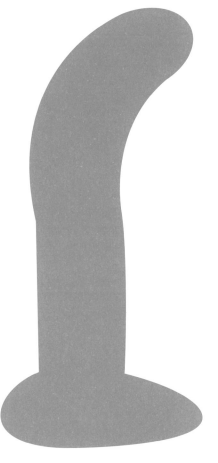

Tantus Slow Drive dildo

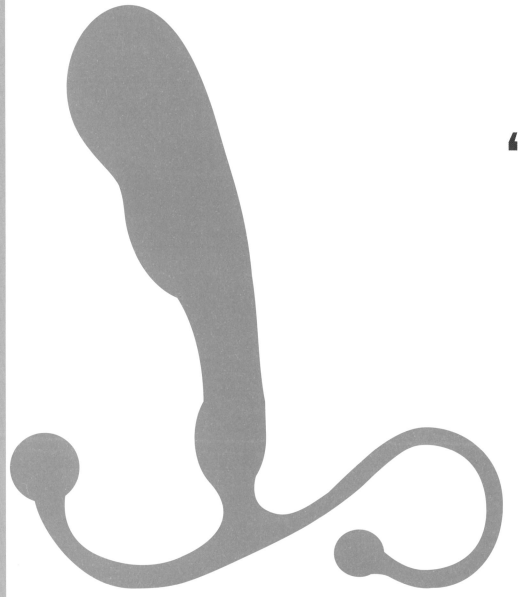

Aneros Helix Syn prostate massager

FROM OUR SURVEY

" *Wow, was it ever magical! After about 5 minutes of tickling the Ida against the outside with a rotation, she had the toy lubed up and it was already up to its neck inside me! The rotation was wild and wonderful, and the settings really were something shocking. . . . I laughed, I laughed some more, and then I nearly screamed! She was giving me oral sex while going through the various throbbing vibration settings on the toy, and I was on cloud nine. I was semi-erect, but it was just too much stimulation for my pelvic region to process. I was being penetrated, vibrated, stroked, and sucked. Glory, glory hallelujah.* "

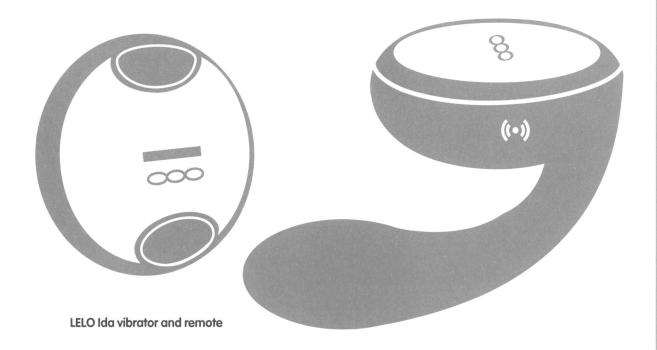

LELO Ida vibrator and remote

perceives and rewards difference, so when a sound or sensation remains the same for a while, it'll ignore that stimulus so that it can focus on new ones. And as with life, so with vibrators. If you leave your vibrator in one spot for too long, your nerve endings will stop responding. But as long as you continue to move it—even slightly—your body will stay sensitive to pleasure. That's why it's better to turn the vibration off and on from time to time, move it around, or use vibration on a dildo instead of placing the vibrator directly in or against your anus.

Prostate-specific toys. As toys for men, and for prostate play in particular, have become more acceptable and widespread, tons of prostate-specific toys have hit the market. The Aneros was originally designed as a therapeutic device for solo prostate massage; it's specially designed to press against the prostate with each squeeze of the sphincter muscles, an action that can promote prostate health. When the Aneros came along, it quickly gained notoriety as a fabulous way to enjoy hands-free pleasure as well. Since then, many imitations have been produced, plus a whole heap of other curved prostate toys.

Inflatable toys. Shaped like dildos or butt plugs, these toys are usually firm enough to insert into your butt before you inflate them. Once the toy is inside, it can be inflated using the handheld pump that's attached to it. In this way, the sphincter muscles and rectum are spread open as the toy slowly increases in size. (Some inflatable butt plugs even have a vibration option.) Some people like to use them as a way to "train" their sphincters to open wider. Bonus: an inflatable toy is many different sizes all at once, depending how much you inflate it. It's like having multiple toys in one!

Anal hooks and cock rings. Bondage and butt plugs—they're a natural match! Don't be put off by the name *anal hooks*; they are so much more pleasurable than they sound. They're curved metal hooks with a ball on one end that rests inside the butt, and the outer "handle" can be attached to a rope or other restraints. When you move even slightly, the metal hook moves, too, delivering subtle pleasure to the anus (and to the prostate, if you've got one). The cock ring and plug work in a similar way. The ring goes around the base of the penis and testicles, while the ball is inserted into the anus. And you don't have to save your set for sexual encounters. You can wear your cock-ring-cum-plug while you're at work, while you're dancing, or even when you're riding a motorcycle! (Quick safety note: metal cock rings are not recommended for beginners. If the wearer gets erect but can't ejaculate or go soft in another way, a trip to the emergency room will be next on the agenda. So if you're a first-timer, go for flexible cock rings that don't come with anal attachments, because they can be put on and taken off easily, whether you're hard or soft.)

FROM OUR SURVEY

When I flexed my sphincters, I got a great prostate massage [from the Doc Johnson OptiMALE prostate massager]. The texture was nice; the size was just right.

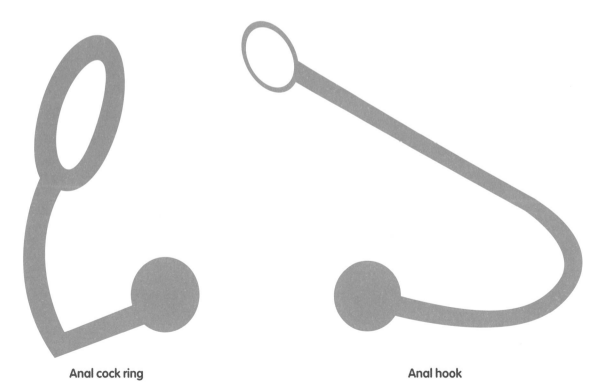

Anal cock ring

Anal hook

TOY FEATURES

Now that you're au fait with some of the options, here's what to keep in mind when you buy—and the same applies if you're reappropriating another sex toy or other object for anal use. Make sure your toy has these five characteristics:

1. Flared base. Very important! Everything you put into your butt needs to be shaped in such a way that it won't get swallowed up, so to speak, as you play. Use a butt plug with a flared base or a string of anal beads with a ring at one end—something that's solid and wide enough to let you pull the toy out easily. A vibrating egg with the battery pack on the outside, for instance, isn't a good choice because the wire might snap when you pull the toy out. That means—you guessed it—a trip to the emergency room (and a broken vibrator, to add insult to injury!).

2. Smooth texture. Be sure that your anal toy is smooth, with no rough edges. Some plastic toys have rough seams where the two sides of the toy meet. Watch out for these since they can tear the sensitive rectal lining.

3. Easy to clean. Using an anal toy with a nonporous surface means you can rest assured your toy is actually thoroughly clean after washing it. It's okay to sterilize your toy by boiling it (see page 134 to find out how), but be sure your toy is made of a material that won't be destroyed by the heat, and never boil anything that has a motor in it. Stick to this maxim: When in doubt, cover your toy with a condom before use.

4. Flexible. If it's deeper or faster play you're after, make sure that your toy can handle your rectum's twists and turns. It should bend easily and shouldn't poke or jab you as you play.

5. Unbreakable. While your toy should definitely be flexible, be sure it's durable, too. You don't want it to break when it's inside of you.

CLEANING YOUR ANAL TOYS

Soap and water are all it takes to clean nonporous toys for your own use (or for use with a partner with whom you're fluid-bonded). For porous toys, you may need something more thorough than soap to be totally safe and avoid infection. There's no need to use harsh chemicals: boiling your toy or using a condom on it will do the trick. If you're using soap, you don't need to buy a special kind, because regular soap is antibacterial by nature (that's why we use it!). You can also use a standard toy cleaner. Lather up your toy for at least 15 seconds. And, unless your toy is made of metal, wood, glass, or plastic, make sure your soap is free from oil or added moisturizing creams. Many soaps these days contain moisturizers; they might feel lovely on your hands, but they can destroy the finish on your toy.

For more thorough cleaning—especially if you're sharing your toys—you can boil silicone, metal, or borosilicate glass toys (without mechanical bits). Boiling your toys for at least 3 minutes will kill any E. coli, parasites, and STIs. (Just beware of the temperature of your toy after you boil it; you may need to let it cool down a little before resuming play.)

Some people like to disinfect their toys by soaking them in a solution of one part bleach to nine parts water, povidine iodine (Betadine), or hydrogen peroxide (full strength) for 20 minutes—but exposing your toy to these chemicals might destroy it, especially if it's made from a natural material like wood. And there's really no need to go to all that trouble anyway. The absolute easiest way to keep your toys clean is to use a condom every time and to remove and discard the condom when you're done. Toys don't need fancy, ultra-sensitive condoms, so just get the thick, reliable, cheap ones. Your toys won't notice the difference!

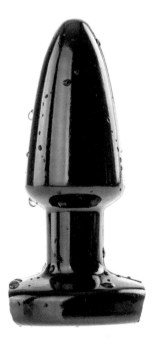

STRAPPING IT ON

A strap-on harness can be a super-fabulous, empowering tool. While harnesses are usually worn by people who haven't got penises, they can actually be worn by anyone—for instance, by a person whose penis doesn't always stay erect, by someone who wants to penetrate a partner post-ejaculation, or by someone who simply doesn't want to use a penis for penetration. If you've already got a penis, you'll be able to buy a penis-friendly style of harness featuring a pouch for holding your package—or you can use just about any two-strap or thigh harness. There are also harnesses that let you add a dildo above your package, which enables you to penetrate two holes at once.

Regardless of your sex, gender, and motives, using a strap-on can be incredibly hot, and it can be a fun experience for both giver and receiver. The giver might feel strong and powerful, partly because of the power that society bestows upon the Almighty Penis—and that can hold true whether or not the giver already has a cock. After all, it can be really exciting to have a penis at your disposal that's always hard, obedient, and ready to go! In fact, a woman I know actually used her harness when she was renegotiating her mortgage over the phone. She strapped on the biggest dildo she could find before she made the call—and it gave her the extra boost of confidence she needed to negotiate without backing down.

Some couples love engaging in sexual role reversal—that is, when the partner who's usually the active penetrator takes the receptive role for a change. For some folks, donning a dildo is a sexy expression of masculine energy; for others, embodying both gender expressions in a single body is a major turn-on. Still others love it when a "feminine" partner takes an active role during penetration instead of a passive one. And some people simply love harnesses for their practicality; it's an easy way to penetrate a partner while leaving your hands free so that you can do other fun things with your fingers at the same time.

If you're not used to being the penetrator, strapping on a dildo can be a fun challenge. Once you've got it on, what to do with it might seem pretty obvious—but it can actually be a hard skill to master! Here's a tip: the thrusting action can be achieved through a very subtle tilt of the hips. If you try to move your whole body forward and backward, you're going to get tired awfully quick. A little practice will help you find your own rhythm.

Choosing a harness

As with any other toy, selecting a harness is a personal choice—but here are a few considerations to keep in mind when you're choosing one.

Control. Having a cock that stays in place instead of one that moves across your pelvis can make a big difference in your experience. A harness that stays put and holds your dildo where you want it can make you a more confident, effective lover.

Style. Two-strap, one-strap, or thigh? It's up to you. A **two-strap harness** has, well, two straps, which go between your legs and then separate at your rear. The straps can often be neatly tucked into the folds between each thigh and buttock. This positioning anchors the harness in place. The two straps at the front can be placed on either side of a vulva or penis and testicles to allow easy access to that area during sex.

A **one-strap harness** has a single strap that goes straight down the middle of your body, over your genitals, and up the crack of your butt. This style does offer a little more control—but not enough to make it worthwhile if you can't stand butt floss. If you like wearing G-string underwear, though, you might really like this type of harness. Plus, the single strap can also hold a vaginal or anal toy in place. (People with penises don't usually find one-straps as comfortable as two-strap harnesses.)

FROM OUR SURVEY

I like the look of my Aslan Jaguar. It feels feminine, and I like the way it feels on my skin. It's comfortable and adjustable, and it's fairly easy to get in and out of. I like that my harness has two straps so my bits are accessible.

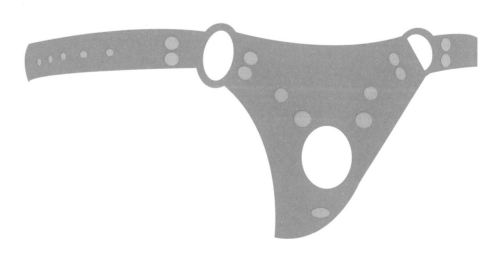

FROM OUR SURVEY

"I never thought about using a thigh harness until I had a hysterectomy and couldn't use my usual harness for several weeks. I reluctantly resigned myself to using a thigh harness—but then I rarely ever went back to my two-strap. The thigh harness gave me amazing control, and I loved cuddling with my partner while fucking her anally."

Thigh harnesses are highly underrated. Just about everyone finds them easy to use. But because of the dildo's odd position on the thigh, many people don't find them very sexy or realistic. If you can get past that, it might be a good option for you if you aren't into simulating a "real" penis, if your tummy hangs over your pubic bone in the place where a dildo would usually sit, if you're pregnant, or if you have back problems. Plus, you can enjoy more full-body contact during intercourse when you're using a thigh harness—and it's easier to achieve powerful thrusting. And since you have *two* thighs, you could always strap a harness to each and penetrate two partners at the same time!

What's my harness made of?

Leather is the most popular option. Lots of people love the look, feel, and smell of a leather strap-on. But you've got plenty of other choices, too.

Rubber works well. It's vegan, it minimizes friction, and it's easy to clean. (It's also waterproof, of course, so you can even use it in the shower!)

Then there's **cloth**, which is comfortable and practical. You can wear it for hours and then toss it in the wash when you're done. And cloth harnesses have an elastic flexibility that's both a pro and a con. On one hand, the dildo is more likely to move around during use, giving the wearer less control (especially when thrusting at steep angles)—but on the other, the dildo's movement can stimulate the wearer's pubic bone and clitoris, delivering a little frisson of pleasure with each thrust.

FROM OUR SURVEY

Strap it on snug to the hips, and use your upper legs and pelvis; make sure that the dildo is snug. Start with pleasure on the outside to give you time to connect to it. You need to be at one with the dildo as an extension of yourself. If you are not in the moment with the dildo, you may as well be walking the dog.

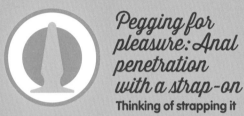

Pegging for pleasure: Anal penetration with a strap-on

Thinking of strapping it on for a session of pegging? Knowing how to work your strap-on with sensuality and confidence is essential to giving your partner the orgasmic pleasure. Here is what you need to know to get started.

Choose your harness: A harness that fits comfortably keeps the dildo secure in different positions without having to hold it in place, and is easy to put on remove and clean. If you have to hold on to your dildo to keep it in place during strap-on sex, your harness is not fully functional. Check out ASLANLeather.com for a complete line of fully functional dildo harnesses.

Choose your dildo: Start with a size that feels comfortable. A smoother dildo is always more comfortable than a textured one. A smaller dildo can provide more direct prostate stimulation and can give you both a chance to experiment with the speed and intensity of your thrusts. Don't be disappointed if you cannot take that 8-inch (20-cm) dick your first time getting pegged. You can train your anal muscles to accept larger and longer cocks over time.

Get to know your tool: Putting on a strap-on for the first time can be equally empowering and awkward. To get comfortable with your new toy, try the harness and dildo on by yourself. Check yourself out in the mirror. See how it moves when you walk. Hold the dildo firmly in your hand, and see how it feels when you press it up against your crotch. Experiment with power dynamics by having your partner suck on your dildo. Chances are you will be excited with all the possibilities that strap-on sex has to offer.

Talk about sex: Get yourselves turned on. A key element of pegging is communication. As the pegger, you are at a disadvantage because you cannot directly feel the effects of the dildo in your partner's ass. You must have open and constant communication with your bottom. Having a lot of dialogue around the play can really intensify the amount of immediate engagement that one or both partners have invested in the play. The more sexy the dialogue, the hotter both partners feel. Exploring your dirty fantasies during sex can be very liberating.

Position: The best position is with the pegger standing and the receiver bent over a counter/couch/bed/chair back at a little lower than hip height.

Let the fun begin: Have lots of lube, gloves, and condoms at hand. Warm up your play area—your partner's anus and surrounding butt cheek area—with your tongue, fingers, or a combination of the two. As your partner becomes more vocal about his or her pleasure, introduce your head with a good amount of lube and press it against the hole gently until you see the sphincter begin to respond by expanding. Once you have entered, go slowly and get your partner to let you know how it feels. If your partner feels discomfort, slowly pull out and play some more until you both feel ready to try again. Anal penetration can take some time to adjust to, so be patient. You may have to try a few times before your partner can fully accept your cock.

Once you are in, remember that you do not have to completely insert your cock. You can keep your hand at the base to shorten the length if necessary. Experiment with your thrust length and speed to see what feels good.

When you are both comfortable with the pegging process, you can expand your repertoire of positions and graduate to being experienced peggers!

—From Carey Gray, owner of ASLANleather.com

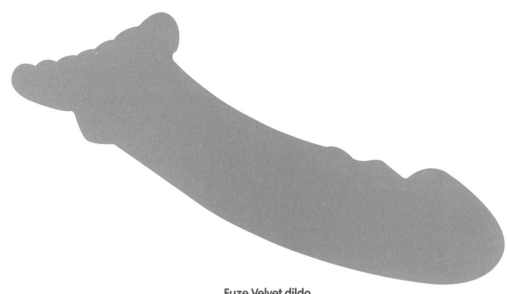

Fuze Velvet dildo

Harness the pleasure

The biggest complaint I hear from folks who wear strap-ons is that they want to experience more pleasure themselves while they play. The receiver gets plenty of stimulation from the dildo's thrusts, but aside from the (very real!) psychological pleasure of penetrating a partner, the wearer might feel a bit shortchanged on sensation. If you have a vagina, try using a dildo with balls or ribs that hang down over the clitoris and can stimulate the clit with each thrust. A vibrating dildo can give added pleasure, too, especially for the receiver, but it usually numbs out the wearer, unfortunately. A remote-controlled toy, like the We-Vibe, is a better choice. It sits against the clit and inside the vagina, and you can control the vibes so that you won't become numb to the pleasure. And it's so small and thin that a dildo can sit over it quite comfortably.

Double-ended dildos can also provide pleasure à deux, either with or without a harness. They've got two heads and usually have a gentle *V* shape. The smaller end penetrates the wearer, and the longer end, which sticks out like an erect penis, penetrates the receiver. Some people love them, but they do have disadvantages. The piece that penetrates the wearer may be too large or small, or the external part might not be as perky because of the way the toy sits inside the wearer's body.

Alternatively, if you're wearing the harness, you can also wear a butt plug (or vaginal plug) for added stimulation. It'll be held in place by the leg strap or straps.

FROM OUR SURVEY

The Fuze Velvet is a wonderful size for double penetration. I like the textured base of this dildo—feels lovely against the clit, and ass, too! Love the control and pleasure for my own clit when I put it in a harness.

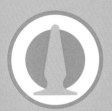

Safer sex is hotter sex

Especially when you know how to put on a condom with your mouth! Suck the tip between your lips (but don't chew) and place the tip of the condom against the penis or toy. Push the condom over the head of the penis with your lips pursed tightly. Once the condom has covered the head, use your hands to unroll it the rest of the way down while your mouth bobs up and down as you work. (Of course, if it's easy for you to push the condom all the way down to the base of the penis with your mouth, go for it!)

Using safer-sex supplies is so important. (Review the section on STIs in chapter 3 to remind yourself why!) And if you're enjoying anal play, you'll want to have plenty of condoms on hand to cover penises or toys. Always use condoms that have been stored at reasonable temperatures (neither too hot nor too cold), check their expiration dates, be sure the packet is free from punctures or tears, and never open a condom packet with your teeth! Finally, remember to avoid condoms or lubes with spermicide or nonoxynol-9. These harsh chemicals can cause irritation or tearing of sensitive tissues, making STI transmission more likely.

CONDOM SENSE

This might seem like old news for most of us, but a refresher course can't hurt! Here's the right way to use a condom:

1. Put a dime-sized dollop of lubricant inside the tip of the condom. It'll increase the pleasure for the penis and will prevent friction.

2. Pinch the air out of the tip of the condom.

3. Place the condom over the tip of the penis, with the roll on the outside (so that the condom looks like a sombrero).

4. Roll the condom over the penis to its base.

5. Hold the base of the condom while you pull out after ejaculation—and you should always pull out after ejaculation, whether you're finished having sex or not.

6. Pull the condom off from the tip of the penis as you hold the base with your other hand. (Otherwise, the ejaculate could spill everywhere.)

7. Put the used condom in the trash, not the toilet.

Condoms can be a little trickier if you're uncircumcised. Here's the best way to put a condom on a penis with a foreskin: Roll the foreskin down; then, put the condom on, and roll it down just past the head of the penis. Hold the condom in place while the foreskin returns to its natural position. Roll the condom down to the base of the penis, and proceed as above. Condoms with larger heads are best for uncircumcised penises, as they have extra room that'll allow the skin to move more freely.

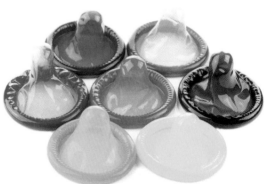

"The 'female condom' is absolutely and positively one of the best condoms in the world! It's virtually indestructible, it's easy to put on, and it's not nearly as invasive as some people say it is. The 'squishy' sound it makes while fucking can be a little off-putting, but it's well worth it! I have a very large penis, and I've actually used the female condom as a regular condom. . . . I just roll it onto my erection, and [use it that way]."

Finding the right condom for you and your partner

Does it surprise you to learn that not all condoms are created equally? It's true! And since condoms are more likely to break during anal play because there's less natural lubrication in the anus than in the vagina (and because sphincter muscles are tighter than most vaginas), it's especially important to get the right size and fit. To do that, you might have to shop around a bit. For one thing, size matters when it comes to condoms. You don't want one that's loose or baggy—but you don't want one that's too tight or constricting, either. So how do you get a sense of the size that's best for you? Luckybloke.com recommends the universal toilet paper roll test. Put your erect penis inside an (empty!) toilet paper roll. If there's extra room, you might be a size small. If the fit is just right, you're probably a medium. And if it feels tight or it's impossible to insert your penis at all, then you're a large.

Then there's shape and texture. Some penises like condoms with roomy heads, while others prefer condoms that are straight from base to tip. Maybe you're a big fan of textured condoms. Some folks swear by them, while others find all those little bumps irritating, especially for anal play. The only way to find out is to experiment!

You might also want to think about what your condoms are made of, especially if you've got a latex allergy. Happily, there are plenty of great non-latex alternatives available. Polyethylene, polyisoprene, and polyurethane are often used in place of latex in condoms. In fact, some people who don't have latex sensitivities still prefer condoms made from these materials. Some of them can be used with oil-based lubricants, unlike their latex counterparts, and many latex-free options seem to transmit body heat more effectively, making them feel more natural during sex. If the price isn't an issue, you might also try lambskin condoms—though they're up to six times as expensive as regular ones. Lambskin condoms contain no latex, and some people find that the natural membrane allows for higher sensation levels than most condoms. Their main disadvantage, though, is that they don't prevent STIs. The thin membrane can contain sperm, but not viruses and bacteria. So if STI protection is one of the reasons you use condoms, then lambskin condoms aren't the right choice for you.

And what if you're a vegan? Vegans avoid using animal products in any form, and an animal protein called casein turns up in the manufacturing processes for most condoms. That's a problem. Luckily, there are lots of animal-free options on the market these days, like products by Sir Richard's Condom Company, Glyde Condoms, and Kimono, including latex-free versions. That's good news for those of us who want to support animal rights—even during sex!

Insertive condoms

Officially called female condoms, insertive condoms are great anal sex accessories. Rumor has it that the insertive condom was actually designed for anal sex in the first place—but the US Food and Drug Administration (USFDA) refused to approve a device intended for use during an illegal act. (That's right: until 2003, anal sex was illegal in many US states.) Today, it's sold in many countries under a variety of brands and names, and it's often referred to as a female condom (FC) or an insertive condom in order to be as inclusive as possible. These are wide condoms that are inserted into a vagina or anus rather than fitting over a penis or toy.

Why use an insertive condom instead of a garden-variety "male" condom? First of all, most insertive condoms are non-latex and are therefore compatible with oil-based lubricants. Second, it's great if you or your partner have trouble maintaining an erection with a condom on, since it's not as tight or constrictive as a standard condoms and because it allows the penetrator's erection to come and go without having to reapply a condom each time. It also reduces the risk that's incurred when you move a penis or toy from the anus to the vagina or mouth. Because the penis or toy shouldn't come into contact with fecal matter when an insertive condom is in place, a partner could move back and forth between anus and vagina or anus and mouth with a lower risk of transmitting harmful bacteria to the vagina, urethra, or mouth.

And that's not all. Since an insertive condom is essentially a plastic tunnel with a cap on one end, the lube you apply before sex will actually stay in place, instead of getting lost in the rectum—and that means maximum pleasure. Plus, you won't have to worry about seeing bits of fecal matter on a penis, finger, or toy since anything you insert will only come into contact with the clean plastic. (You might see some on the outside of the condom when you take it out, but you can do that in private after play is finished.) Finally, insertive condoms are great for anal sex because of the way in which they line the rectum. The receiver gets to experience all the pleasure with far less friction and minimal discomfort. With intercourse with a regular male condom or no condom, any bits of fecal matter in the rectum get rubbed around, similar to getting a massage when there is sand stuck in the massage oil. The FC acts like a barrier—as though you had plastic wrap over your back so that the bits of sand did not constantly rub your skin but you could still feel the pleasure of the hand movements. Similarly, the bits of matter in your butt remain in place with the FC over the top of them, buffering the rectum from being irritated by each thrust. In addition, the rectum does not get potentially irritated by the rubber friction of the condom going in and out—a win-win either way!

So why isn't everyone singing the praises of the insertive condom? Well, for one thing, change can be tough. The insertive condom doesn't look like a standard condom, so it might take some time to get used to it—and some people aren't turned on by the sight of a vulva or anus with a plastic ring hanging out of it. Also, it makes a sort of "rubbing" sound during sex, which is a turnoff for some folks. Since it's a finite length, it limits the depth of penetration, and it's more expensive than conventional condoms—although one study found that washing and drying them carefully up to seven times still maintained the integrity of the condom. You certainly can't do that with standard condoms!

It's completely up to you to decide which type of condom is best for you and your partner—but do consider giving insertive condoms a chance during anal before you write them off. You might be very pleasantly surprised!

Gloves

Like any other part of the body, hands can transfer bacteria, such as E. coli, as well as other infections from one part of the body to another or from one person to another. That's why it's important to use them for anal play, especially if you have cuts or open sores on your hands. If you're not sure whether you have cuts on your hands, or whether an older cut has healed, try this simple test: Put a few drops of lemon juice or alcohol on your hands. Does it sting? If so, the cut is open, and it's a standing invitation to STIs such as HIV. Cover your hands with disposable gloves before anal play to protect yourself.

Apart from STI concerns, lots of folks like using gloves for anal play because they make cleanup so easy. If you want to switch from anal to other types of play mid-sex, or if you just want to stop sex altogether, a glove comes off quickly and makes the transition simple—it's far more convenient than getting up to wash your hands, and it's more effective than using a baby wipe.

Gloves should fit snugly; they shouldn't be so tight that they cut off your circulation, but they should be tight enough for you to be able to feel through the glove. Latex gloves are ideal because they stretch nicely, but many folks have latex allergies to consider. Vinyl is latex-free, but it's not as stretchy, so vinyl gloves won't fit as well as latex. Try gloves made from nitrile, a synthetic, latex-free rubber with good stretch and excellent strength. Nitrile gloves are often compatible with oil-based lubricants as well. You'll find that some gloves (latex, usually) have a powder in them to make them easier to put on. If the powder irritates you, though, just go for powder-free ones.

And you don't have to stick to boring beige gloves, either. They come in lots of colors—green, pink, blue, and black. Personally, I love black gloves for the same reason I like anal toys that are black: they camouflage any bits of poop that might get stuck on them. (Besides, the black ones are a little sexier, and they're more likely to match whatever you're wearing!)

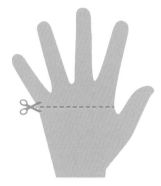

Making a dental dam out of a glove

Dental dams

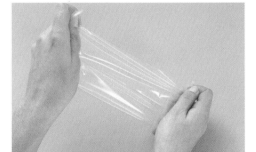

Dental dams are thin sheets of latex that prevent the transmission of STIs, usually when you're giving or receiving oral pleasure. There are latex-free options available as well. But they're great for all sorts of anal play, too: some folks use dental dams specifically for STI prevention, while others love them simply because they're more comfortable when they feel clean. If you're in a pinch and you haven't got dental dams on hand, try using plastic wrap instead. You can also cut a condom up the side, from base to tip, and spread it out. Alternatively, cut a (non-powdered) glove into a custom size; the thumb-hole is handy since it can easily be tucked inside the butt.

Lubricant

I've said it before, and I'll say it again: Lube is absolutely critical to pleasurable anal play. The rectum has a mucosal lining—that is, it's got a small amount of natural lubrication—but not enough to prevent uncomfortable friction. And if you're using a condom over a sex toy or penis, you'll need even more lube to make anal play pleasurable. What all this means is that a good lube can make the difference between pleasure and pain during penetration.

Each person has individual preferences when it comes to lube, so you might need to experiment a bit to find the one that works best for you. The lube you use for other kinds of play might suit your anal adventures, or you may want to reserve another type of lube specifically for anal play. Some folks even concoct their own recipes for lube combinations: one part of this type, two parts of that one, and a dash of a third to ensure optimal glide. In general, though, most anal aficionados prefer thicker lubes because they stay in place more effectively than thinner ones, which often get pushed deeper and deeper into the rectum during sex. It might even be a good idea to coat the anal and rectal walls with a thick lube and then put a thinner version on any toys, fingers, or penises you plan to insert. That way, the toy or penis will glide smoothly over the thick lube inside. This strategy helps lubes stay put, makes play more pleasurable, and minimizes interruptions to play (you won't have to stop as often to reapply your favorite lube!).

Another tip is to choose a bottle of lube that has a pump, which makes for easy application when you're working with only one hand. (One-handed lube application is especially important for keeping the bottle—and one of your hands—clean.) You might also consider investing in a lube shooter. It's a handy tool that's used like a syringe. Fill it with your lube of choice, add some more lube to the tip, and then shoot the contents up your butt. It's a great way to fast-track the lube to all the right places even before a finger or toy goes in.

Water-based lubes are the most common. They're water-soluble and safe to use with all types of toys, but they're not as long-lasting as silicone- or oil-based varieties, as the water in them evaporates with friction and exposure to air. (These lubes can be rehydrated with a spritz of water, though. If you don't want to add more lube, you can just spray some water on the area to make it slippery again.)

What's in your water-based lube besides water? Glycerin, possibly. Whether it's derived from animal or vegetable fats, glycerin acts like a sugar, which means it feels sticky when it dries out. Many folks dislike that sensation, so they avoid lubes with glycerin. Plus, glycerin acts as a suppository—that is, it encourages BMs—and that's not the desired outcome during anal play for most people! Flavored lubes contain glycerin to make them tasty, but they're not recommended for anal play because they dry out quickly and get very sticky. (If you do want to add some flavor to your oral-anal romps, use a little dab of flavored lube externally. When you move to internal play, switch to a glycerin-free lube.)

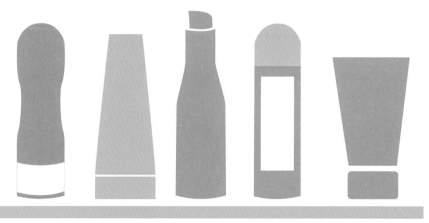
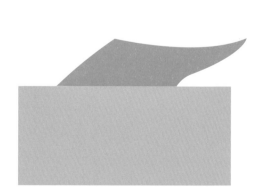

Some water-based lubes contain parabens. These preservatives turn up in lots of body-care products and appear under various names, such as methylparaben. Take care—parabens have been linked to cancer in some studies, so lots of people prefer to avoid lubes that contain them. Always familiarize yourself with the ingredients in your lube before you use it.

Healthier lubricant ingredients include carrageenan, a seaweed extract that's been used as a food additive for hundreds of years. These days, scientific studies are investigating its potential as an HPV inhibitor. Aloe vera also pops up in many eco-friendly body-care products these days. It's nice and thick, acts as a natural moisturizer, and generally feels great on the skin.

Silicone lubes are longer lasting than their water-based counterparts because they don't contain water, which will evaporate, and because silicone can't be absorbed by skin or by mucous membranes. That means they won't dry out like water-based lubes, so you won't need to reapply them again and again. They feel very silky, even when they're only used for external play. There's just one drawback, though: silicone-based lubricants aren't compatible with some silicone toys. Whether or not a toy and a silicone-based lube will work well together depends on the quality of the lube and the quality of the toy. Here's how to find out: Test a little of the lube on an inconspicuous part of your toy. If it feels tacky or starts to discolor within 1 minute, the toy and lube aren't compatible. Try Pjur Original, an odorless, tasteless silicone

lubricant that works with many better-quality silicone toys. Or try a water-based lube with just a hint of silicone; this type of lube seems to be more compatible with silicone toys.

The good news is, silicone lubes are compatible with all types of condoms, and they're unlikely to irritate sensitive skin. Oddly, silicone lubes tend to be less reactive than many "natural" lubes. And they even stay in place underwater, so they're great for use in the shower, tub, or Jacuzzi. But watch out for spilled lube, because that super-slippery quality that makes it so awesome during sex also means that it can be dangerous in the wrong places. If you spill silicone lube on the floor or in the shower, clean it up with soap and water immediately, or you could slip and fall.

Oil-based lubes have incredible staying power, feel natural, and are widely available. Use coconut oil, walnut oil, grapeseed oil, and even olive oil—but do avoid non-food-grade oils, such as baby oil or mineral oil. Remember that the rectum is highly absorbent, so stay away from oil-based lubes with perfumes and other synthetic ingredients. Look at it this way: if you wouldn't put it in your mouth, don't put it up your butt!

Oil does have its limitations. It can be used with wood, glass, or metal toys, but it can't be used with latex, elastomer, or silicone. Like silicone-based lubes, oil-based lubes are incredibly slippery, so be sure to clean up any spills with soap and water. Although oils can be used with polyurethane and nitrite condoms, they can't be used with latex condoms. (Latex gloves are thicker and won't break down as easily, so you can use them with oil-based lubes for up to 15 minutes.)

Watch out for the numbing agents that appear in some anal lubes. They're designed to desensitize the anal area to prevent pain during anal play. Some folks reach for these lubes because their experiences have taught them that anal sex is painful. And, yes, it might hurt if you're penetrated quickly by something large, like a penis or toy, without a proper warm-up. But you already know that anal sex doesn't have to be painful if you proceed slowly and listen to your body, so there's really no need to use a numbing lube.

By now, you hopefully have all the information you need to choose the best tools for the job—from toys to safe-sex supplies. You've got plenty of positions to choose from. But don't forget that taking care of your partner after sex is as important as being prepared before you begin. Read on for tips for taking care of your partner's emotional and physical needs post-sex.

Chapter 9
AFTERCARE:
ADDRESSING POST-SEX EMOTIONAL AND PHYSICAL NEEDS

You've just had a great anal sex session, and now it's time to move on to other activities, like sleeping, going to work, doing chores, picking up the kids, or making dinner. But before you get up and go, it's important to devote a little bit of space to post-sex aftercare to help you process your anal adventures. Paying attention to a few key details—either immediately after sex or after you've gotten some sleep or rest—can make for a smooth transition to your post-anal-sex life, both physically and emotionally. This chapter will show you how to simplify cleanup after anal, how to nourish and restore your body after sex, why practical post-sex communication is a must, and how to create space for the emotions that tend to be roused by anal sex.

FROM OUR SURVEY

" My aftercare generally involves cuddles, lots of water, baby wipes, and comfy clothing." And don't assume that aftercare is limited to the partner or partners who've been penetrated. The penetrator also has psychological needs, and emotional surprises may arise for her or him as well. Make sure that everyone has a chance to share, to be heard, and to feel accepted. "

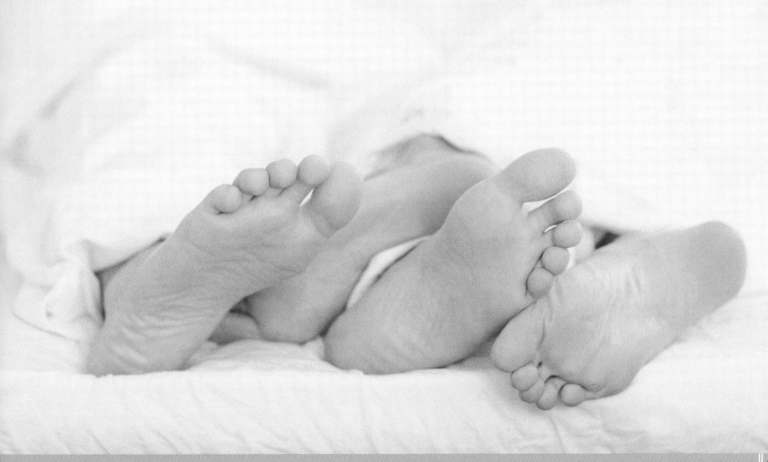

NO-FUSS CLEANUP

This is probably old news to you by now, but here's a quick recap of fast, sanitary cleanup techniques. First, put disposable items, like condoms, paper towels, or baby wipes, in the garbage immediately. Then, gather all of your toys in a towel or large pot. Wash your toys with soap and water and sterilize them (if possible), either right away or within a few hours. If you're using a towel, wash it thoroughly as soon as possible.

Consider investing in a sex pot for easy cleanup of dirty toys! The concept is simple: If you don't like the idea of cooking pasta in the same pot or saucepan you use to sterilize your sex toys, buy a large pot and keep it in the bedroom (or in another private place where your mom won't stumble across it when she comes over to help you cook). After sex, gather the toys in your sex pot, and then wash or boil them in it après sex. Afterward, both the pot and your toys will be ready for your next anal adventure—and you'll always have your sex pot nearby to chuck used toys into when you're done using them.

And if you're using disposable gloves during anal sex, here's a simple technique that'll help you contain the soiled part of the glove.

Step 1: Pull the cuff of one glove over your whole hand, turning the glove inside out as it comes off. Don't let go of the cuff of the first glove while you move to the next step.

Step 2: Pull the cuff of the second glove over your hand in the same way, drawing it over the first inside-out glove as you pull it off. Now you have a neat package that's relatively clean before it goes into the trash. Done! (Well, there's one more step, actually: always wash your hands right after you finish cleaning up—especially if you're going to continue to touch your or your partner's genital or anal areas.)

FROM OUR SURVEY

I don't like to put sticky, butty, hands on my partners, so I try to clean my hands as soon as possible. Baby wipes are good for that. I also try to wipe the lube off my ass, too. Often, when toys are involved, I just set them aside on a tissue until I have time to clean them later.

FROM OUR SURVEY

" *If you're the person who's been penetrated, don't rush out to a big party or plan on doing a lot of errands afterward, especially if you've taken it deep and hard. You may need to visit the toilet a few times before it feels like things have settled down.* "

PHYSICAL AFTERCARE

The resulting physiological impact of anal sex can be more dramatic than other types of sex. That's not meant to scare you off; it's simply good to know in advance. Here's why: because the anus has minimal natural lubrication, the anal opening might feel sore post-pleasure, especially if you didn't use enough lube. Remember that our bodies have a higher pain tolerance during arousal, so you won't always feel discomfort during sex as much as you might afterward. This isn't to say that you *will* feel pain after anal sex, but after a long session with lots of thrusting or with a toy (or finger) that has ridges and curves, the anal area might feel tender and sensitive. Applying a little aloe vera to the area or relaxing in a warm bath laced with Epsom salts can help soothe inflamed skin.

If you experience bleeding after sex, it may be because you have internal hemorrhoids that were irritated and opened by the activity. Don't worry; this isn't serious, and the best thing to do to fix it is to lie on your tummy and let time and gravity heal the area. Some people like to apply compresses with vitamin E, chamomile, calendula, or ice to help hemorrhoids heal.

Anal bleeding post-sex could also be a result of fissures, which are small tears in the anus's skin. Again, they usually heal on their own, but for any persistent or specific problems, or where bleeding is profuse and/or persists, the best thing to do is seek medical attention.

It's also important to be mindful of a few sexual-health issues. If you have a penis and you've penetrated your partner with it, you may be at risk of a urinary tract infection (UTI) if bacteria from your partner's anus have traveled to your bladder. To prevent UTIs—especially if you didn't use a condom and/or didn't ejaculate—try to urinate within an hour after sex. You want to expel those bacteria before they wreak havoc on your bladder.

If a condom broke during anal play and your partner is or could be HIV-positive, go to the hospital to get a drug cocktail called a post-exposure prophylaxis (PEP). If taken within 72 hours, it can reduce the risk of contracting HIV. And the sooner it's taken after exposure, the more effective it is, so don't wait to seek medical help if you think you've been exposed to HIV. Then, get an HIV test 3 months later. In the meantime, consider

seeing a counselor or therapist, since waiting for a test result can be a serious emotional strain. The reality is that HIV affects all kinds of people, regardless of sexual practices or drug habits, so prevention is the best strategy. PEP is just a backup plan for when an accident does happen.

Finally, do see a doctor if something doesn't feel quite right after sex—whether it's right away or a few days after the fact. There's no shame in telling a medical practitioner that you engaged in anal sex, and the sooner you address any infections or other medical issues, the more quickly they'll heal.

Everyone's body responds differently to anal sex. Some people experience no "side effects" at all, but others do experience constipation after sex. Still others may have a series of BMs over the next couple of hours. This is why many folks time their anal adventures to allow for a couple of hours of downtime afterward, when a bathroom is never far away. That's especially advisable during your first few forays into anal sex, when you're still working out how your body will react to this new form of pleasure.

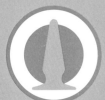

Restore and replenish after anal sex

Your body needs to recover after anal sex, so be sure to give yourself some time before your next session of anal pleasure. How long? Well, if you're a beginner, allow for a couple weeks between encounters—at least until you know your body and its reactions well. This downtime will allow the rectal mucosa to regain their balance, especially if you cleaned yourself out before or after sex. Taking an acidophilus probiotic can help to restore the natural bacteria in your butt. And as always, make sure to drink plenty of water and to eat well to maintain your energy levels.

FROM OUR SURVEY

" Aftercare is checking in, having a conversation, and generally being available to a person who I've enjoyed anal sex with. With a partner, I like to acknowledge any mistakes or awkwardness that might have come up, since I think anal play can be a more vulnerable type of sex. "

PRACTICAL POST-SEX COMMUNICATION

Any new sex adventure is best when followed by an honest, open discussion about what worked, what didn't, and what you'd like to do differently next time. And even if you're not trying anything new, regular debriefing can only make for better sex. (Of course, you don't have to have a discussion after every single sex romp—unless you want to, that is!) As with comedy, so with discussing sex: timing is everything, and the best time for a post-sex check-in is anywhere from a few hours up to a day after the encounter. That's because intense discussions *right* after sex can be a

little tough to swallow when our hearts and bodies are so open—but then again, if you wait too long to talk, you're at risk of forgetting everything you wanted to say. Allowing for a little distance—but not too much—makes it easier for you and your partner to give and receive feedback. If talking about sex with a partner doesn't come naturally to you, review chapter 6 for ways to initiate conversations about your erotic life.

EMOTIONAL AFTERCARE FOR YOU AND YOUR PARTNER

FROM OUR SURVEY

" The only thing that's especially important to me is that my partner remains with me after the session. Once a partner left the room immediately afterward, and I found this quite distressing. "

Any kind of sex can be highly emotional, depending upon the kind of connection you have with your partner, your general stress levels, your history with anal sex, your expectations for the sex session, your partner's experience and reaction, and so much more. And anal sex seems to have a special way of bringing hidden emotions to the surface. Sometimes we're in tune with those emotions—but at other times, they might not appear to make much sense. Many people find that anal play cuts to the core of who we really are, as opposed to the kind of person we'd like to be or how we'd like others to see us. For one thing, all of the taboos discussed in chapter 1 can rear their ugly heads during and after anal play—and that means feelings of shame, "dirtiness," or "unmanliness" can keep you from of lying back and savoring a perfectly natural, pleasurable experience. So, give yourself and your partner time and space to allow these emotions to surface and dissipate. Notice them, voice them, and discuss them—even if you feel shame about feeling shame! That's okay, too.

Also, sometimes you might feel confused by unexpected emotional responses—ones you no longer believe in, or ones you thought were long gone. The fact is, the body can store these emotions in your subconscious for a long time, until they're acknowledged and processed. Emotions are real, and they don't usually go away when we ignore them. On the contrary—they often get bigger and more complicated. Holding back emotions can have detrimental emotional and physical effects and can even make you anal-retentive—both literally and figuratively! Allowing yourself and your partner space to talk about your anal adventures means better, healthier sex for both of you.

Chapter 10

ADVANCED ANAL:
BDSM, SPANKING, RESTRAINTS, AND LOTS MORE

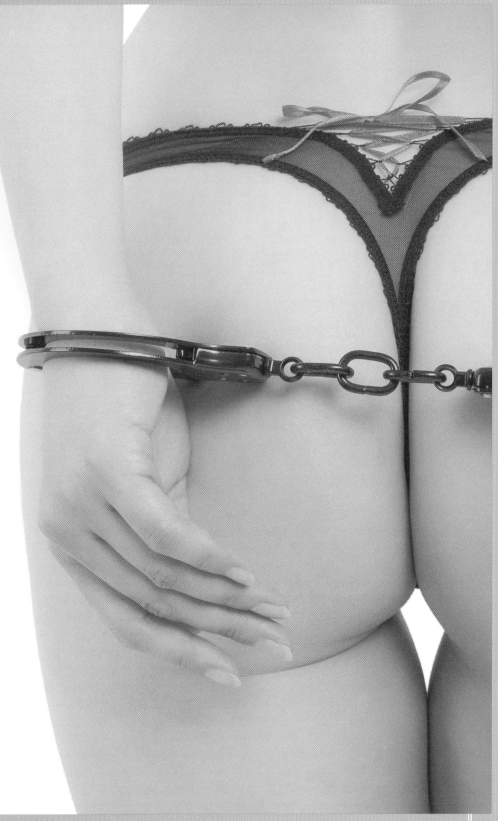

Once you're an experienced anal player, you might be interested in exploring forms of sex that are a little bit edgier. Maybe you're thinking of experimenting with bondage and domination, or maybe having your partner tie you up during anal has always been a secret fantasy of yours. Or maybe you want to include anal play in your regular kink sessions. If you long for deeper, more intense anal play, you might dream of working your way up to fisting, in which four or five fingers are inserted into the anus all at once. Lots of people call these practices kink, but there's no need to get hung up on the word; you don't have to be, or feel, kinky to want to try them on for size. When they're shared between consenting adults, they're perfectly valid forms of sexual expression—just like any other type of sex. So I hope you'll be inspired by this chapter. Think of it as a primer on safe, advanced anal play, from BDSM to double penetration and electrostimulation (it's much sexier than it sounds!) and beyond.

ADVANCED PLAY STARTS WITH GREAT COMMUNICATION

FROM OUR SURVEY

" I got tied up on a bench and spanked by a dominatrix once. She played with my ass and balls while she flogged me and whipped me with about five different kinky objects. Then she played with my ass some more. Good times! "

I can't say it often enough: All kinds of sex require communication and negotiation, and that's even truer when it comes to more advanced, intense sex. This is because some amount of physical and psychological risk accompanies any kind of pleasurable sexual activity. The encounter might not unfold exactly as it was planned, pain may catch you off guard, erections and orgasms don't always happen on demand, and communication errors arise. Just like the rest of life, sex is not always predictable. So when you engage in sex that's more intense, the resulting consequences are generally more intense, too. Disappointment is felt more strongly, the potential for pain is a little higher, and the possibility of miscommunication is greater. That's why it's so important for you and your partner or partners to negotiate desires and boundaries in as much detail as possible. When you're open and communicative about your needs, you'll minimize misunderstandings and errors.

While it's great to be open to experimentation, don't pressure yourself to try lots of new things all at once. For instance, if you're new to anal pleasure and are also curious about double penetration and bondage, by all means try them—but do it one at a time. (Hopefully, there'll be plenty of exciting sex sessions in your future, so you don't need to get through your entire bucket list in a single day!) The reason it's best to limit yourself to one new activity per sex session is that each activity can elicit unforeseen responses, including an awareness of your sexual boundaries—and most of the time, you only know where those boundaries are once you've gone past them. Sometimes that can be exciting and exhilarating, but when several aspects of the encounter are unexpected and uncomfortable, it's harder to process them, and you're less likely to want to try any of the activities again. (Worse still, your relationship with your partner might even suffer from a loss of trust.) Instead, explore each new activity separately, and bring them together only when you have a better understanding of your boundaries, expectations, and desires. Always listen to your gut, and stop when you feel you need to. After all, it's always better to leave the table when you're still a little hungry! That way, you and your partner will be even more excited about the next encounter.

Finally, as with sex of any kind, check in with yourself to be sure that you're actually doing what *you* want to do, and don't feel pressured into an encounter or activity if you're not really into it—even if you've done it a hundred times before. And remember that you can stop what you're doing at any time. What if something feels exciting to you at first but suddenly starts to feel not-so-sexy halfway through? That's completely fine. You're under no obligation to go ahead with it—even if you went to the trouble of hiring a sitter, finding props, and booking a hotel room for the encounter. Give yourself permission to change courses mid-sex or to stop what you're doing altogether.

FROM OUR SURVEY

"Be up front about what you want. Add it as a form of reward, especially in BDSM play—or use it as a punishment, if so desired."

BASIC GUIDELINES FOR ADVANCED ANAL

Folks who engage with more advanced kinds of sex, including anal sex, have developed some generally accepted parameters for BDSM (bondage, dominance, sadism, masochism) play. Here are some of the most important:

Be risk aware

It's vital to know what you're doing before you start to play. Educate yourself on the physical, emotional, and psychological techniques you intend to use, and figure out what's safe for you and your partner. Arguably, sexually speaking, nothing is completely "safe"—except not having sex at all—so you need to be aware of any risks associated with the activities you've chosen and of how to minimize those risks. Have a backup plan in case you are feeling uncomfortable, and know that you can simply sit out this round.

Play sober

Never play when you're intoxicated or high. Be very careful about drinking alcohol at all before play. According to some folks, even one drink is too much, since you want to be alert and aware of your body, of the subtleties of your desires and boundaries, and of the experience of pleasure and pain. You can't make safe choices if you can't think clearly enough to assess risks, to take necessary precautions, and to problem-solve when unintended consequences arise.

Gain consent

Make sure that everyone involved in play is excited and turned on by what you're doing. This means that all parties need to be of legal age, of sound mind, and sober so that they can fully understand the risks associated with the activity you've chosen together. Remember that consent is given of free will, not in exchange for love or from a fear of undesirable alternatives. And it's always temporary; it can be rescinded at any time.

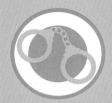

Bondage sessions aren't foolproof

Lots of things can go wrong during bondage encounters, so you need to put safety first. Here's an example of what might go amiss: one of the principles of bondage and restraint is that the person who's tied up should be able to get out of the restraints within 20 seconds. This is why wrist restraints are so popular; they're easy-on, easy-off. Then again, many people love the aesthetic of rope bondage, while others take a more ad hoc approach to the whole thing and use whatever scarves or ties they have lying around. That's okay, but you need to be mindful of the material you're using, and you need to know how to tie it in such a way that it won't cut off your partner's circulation when she or he pulls against it. And you need to have safety equipment on hand—like surgical scissors, for instance. Why? Well, once when I was tied up, I knocked over a lit candle and set the pillow on fire. When things like that happen, you need to be able to get out of your restraints in no more than a few seconds—and that's where scissors come in awfully handy! For details on how to use rope safely and to tie beautifully, see Lord Morpheus' book *Bondage Basics* (2015).

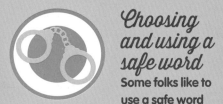

Choosing and using a safe word

Some folks like to use a safe word instead of the word *no* when they want to stop play. That way, you can say no all you like as part of the fun when you actually want things to continue, but you also have a way to call a halt to play when you've truly had enough. One common approach is the traffic-light system: green means "go ahead, all good"; yellow means "slow down, it's getting kind of intense"; and red means "stop *right now*." And this can work for both partners. As a top, even if your partner hasn't called the safe word, you can call your own safe word if you start to feel uncomfortable or if you don't trust your partner's judgment in the moment. (Don't push yourself or your partner outside of your comfort zones; everyone involved deserves to feel great about the pleasure at hand.) Not everyone needs a safe word, though. If it's a game you don't enjoy, just agree that no simply means no.

FROM OUR SURVEY

> *Anything can be kinky, if you think of it that way—or anything is tame, if you think of it like that. It's all down to perspective. For me, anal is just a different kind of sex, like oral sex or hand jobs or dry humping: all forms of sex. But there's more of a release after the buildup of kinky excitement, like spanking or using rope.*

BONDAGE (B)

Restraint can be so exciting. It can be fun to be tied up while other delicious activities are happening—and for some folks, it's the only way they can relax and surrender to the pleasure without feeling guilty about it. Then again, some simply like the physical sensation of being restrained, while still others enjoy the power dynamic that often accompanies the play ("Your butt is mine now!"). It can range from playful ("Don't move while I tantalize your butt!") to intense ("No escaping the butt plug!"). Before experimenting with bondage, though, make sure you're au fait with safety tips. For instance, you should always be sure there's at least a finger's width of room between the restraint and the skin so that blood circulation can carry on as usual. You also need to know which parts of the body can safely be restrained and which can't (like the neck). Never allow yourself to be tied up by someone you don't know well enough to trust. And if you don't feel comfortable with full bondage yet, try holding on to a scarf tied to a bedpost instead. That'll give you a sense of restraint, but you'll be able to let go whenever you want.

DOMINANCE AND SUBMISSION (D/S)

Dominance and submission—the *D* and *S* in BDSM—are about playing with power. In these scenarios, the dominant partner (also known as the top) takes control, while the submissive partner (also known as the bottom) willingly surrenders it for the duration of a scene or a specific period of time. While some people prefer being either a top or a bottom, others are switches who like playing either role. Dominance and submission work well in conjunction with butt play. There are lots of options: the top might take charge of the bottom's anal pleasure or restrict her or him from touching himself or herself or orgasming until permitted. A bottom might be instructed to perform anal play on himself or herself or on a partner, or he or she might be told to give a partner an enema or to bring him or her to multiple orgasms. These are only a few examples, though. The possibilities are infinite! (Just remember that controlling someone who is not turned on by it or who does not consent to surrendering control constitutes abuse.)

FROM OUR SURVEY

" *When I penetrate my partner with anal intercourse, it is the only time I am allowed to orgasm. In receiving anal play, it is a pinnacle of submissive behavior. When my top is properly pleased, anal play is used as a reward.* "

FROM OUR SURVEY

" *Anal is a good way for my dominant partner to assert dominance over me.* "

Power bottoms: Dominance, submission, and anal play

Anal play doesn't have to be about dominance and submission—but they sure do pair well! The potentially thrilling social taboo of anal play, the often intense physical sensation, and the level of trust and vulnerability it takes to engage in safe anal play can easily combine to create a perfect storm of pervy fun. Remember, there's no such thing as an intrinsically dominant or submissive act. You get to decide which acts symbolize which roles to you. Of course you'll negotiate all this ahead of time, making sure that everyone involved gives their enthusiastic consent. Here are some ways to involve D/S in anal play:

• If you enjoy ritual as part of your D/S, the preparation for a butt-play scene can take on deep psychological meaning—whether that means cleaning yourself out or simply laying out the toys and lube.

• If you're a dominant who likes to be anally pleasured, you can instruct your submissive to serve you exactly as you like it (and, perhaps, to clean up afterward, too!).

• For submissives, a butt plug can make even the most unerotic domestic service an experiment in arousal. Butt plugs are great for covert, fully clothed public play, too. The gradual coaxing of a submissive's body to open up to larger and larger anal toys over a period of weeks or months can fulfill "training" fantasies in a big way.

• Anal play also works nicely into D/S-inflected exclusivity arrangements. ("You can play with others, but your ass belongs to me.")

• A dominant might require that their submissive keep their anal region shaved or waxed, or perhaps soft and furry.

• If you're into intense psychological play, anal scenes can give you a way into some big emotions. Mainstream culture tells us anal sex is painful or is only ever a form of punishment. In truth, anal sex should never hurt and should always be fully consensual. But in a fear play or punishment scene, you can play with these misconceptions for emotional impact, such as by "threatening" to tear someone with your big cock or toy or "forcing" someone to accept anal penetration because they've been "bad." Of course you'll really just use the dildo their body can accommodate comfortably.

• Shame is another common emotion the world associates with the anus. After all, it's a dirty, bad place, right? Wrong! But this association can make for a satisfying humiliation scene, if that's your kink. "Only bad girls and dirty boys like it up the ass," or "Lick my butthole, pig!"

• Enema play is a fun option here, too, and pairs especially well with role-play. A stern nurse might need to rinse out a bad patient's bowels if they're not clean enough, for instance. Just make sure to learn how to use an enema properly first—a little goes a long way!

In short, combine your creativity and specific erotic hot buttons with safety knowledge and thorough negotiation, and you can use anal play to enhance D/S dynamics of all kinds.

—From Andrea Zanin,
sex educator and writer,
sexgeek.wordpress.com

SADO-MASOCHISM (S/M)

The term *S and M* is bandied around quite a bit, but what does it actually mean? Here's a working definition: A sadist takes pleasure in inflicting pain on someone *who enjoys receiving pain.* (Inflicting pain on someone who is not turned on by it or who doesn't consent to it is assault.) A masochist, on the other hand, takes pleasure in receiving pain. A sadist is often, but not always, also a dominant, and by the same token, a masochist is often, but not always, also a submissive. That's the joy of sex play: you get to make your own rules and roles, and they can be as fluid as you want them to be. For example, you can be a masochistic dominant who instructs your submissive to spank you hard while receiving anal sex. And you can enjoy S/M play without any power-exchange dynamics, too. All you need to do is ask for a firmer touch rather than a gentle one. You can ask to be flogged or spanked without involving any seizing or surrendering of control too.

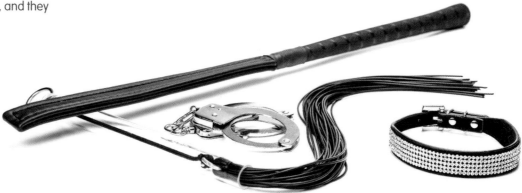

SPANKING

Spanking is an easy addition to the excitement of anal play since the butt is, conveniently, already front and center. Some people love spanking or being spanked because they enjoy feeling dominant or submissive. Others love engaging with the taboo that surrounds spanking—and some folks simply like the physical sensation. Whatever your reasons, spanking can be a great way to make anal play even sexier. Here are a few caveats to keep in mind before you start:

• Never spank when you're angry, even if you enjoy playing with dominance. As with all kink play, spanking is supposed to give pleasure—even if it's painful. Make sure you're calm and relaxed.

• Remove any rings from your hands before you begin.

• Get your partner aroused before spanking him or her. It's much more pleasurable when the endorphins are flowing.

• Start gently and increase the intensity slowly. Don't kick off with the biggest thwack you can muster! As you ramp up the intensity levels, keep things interesting. Alternate between heavy and light smacks. Rub or massage the area in between heavy hits. Keep your partner guessing to enhance the anticipation: will your next touch be a hard smack or a gentle stroke? Count out the spanks as you're administering them—or make the spankee do the counting. There are so many ways to play!

• Watch where you're spanking. Aim for the lower, fleshier part of the butt and the upper thigh. Avoid the lower back and the place where the butt meets the back. Steer clear of the tailbone, spine, and penis. Try different types of slaps—a flat, open hand, a cupped hand, and slaps with toys, like a wooden spoon, flogger, crop, paddle, or even a wet towel. Stay tuned in to your partner's reaction. Pay attention to how his or her butt responds, as well as your partner's breathing and body language in general. Respect your partner when he or she says no or uses the safe word, and don't push any further after that.

"I force myself to wear a butt plug for extended periods of time. It's a fun kind of torture to be stuffed while you go about doing things, and every movement is overstimulating. You just beg for the release of having it out combined with the agonizing need to be screwed."

DOUBLE PENETRATION

Traditionally, double penetration involves two penises: one inside the bottom's vagina, and one inside the bottom's—well, bottom. But the fact is, penises are completely optional. You can also use two dildos, strap-ons, plugs, fingers or any combination of these. Before you start, you'll want to do plenty of warm-up, starting with clitoral and vaginal/innie play and progressing to anal stimulation. Once you or your partner is ready to go, reserve the smaller penis or toy for the butthole, since most vaginas open more easily than anuses. Here's the easiest position if you're using two penises or strap-ons: The bottom should mount one of the tops for vaginal/innie penetration. Then, the second top squats over both people (getting a good thigh workout in the process!) and penetrates the bottom anally. From there, the bottom can leave both penises or objects inside and move one or both in and out, or the bottom can alternate and insert one while the other exits. Each has its own intensity. And remember that the anal and vaginal openings are very close to one another, and filling one often means that the other can't expand as much as it usually does. That's why it's a good idea to start with smaller toys when you're playing with both openings at once for the first time.

ANAL TRAINING

In the same way that you need to do a few long-distance runs before you attempt a marathon, some folks like wearing a butt plug outside of the bedroom so that their butts become accustomed to the width of the toy or in order to relax into larger butt plugs. Sometimes, it's used as a type of bondage or as a source of undercover pleasure (only the wearer—and her or his partner, perhaps—will know what's going on in the back door!). Alternatively, a plug might be worn to an event or en route to the play space so that the wearer's anus slowly becomes relaxed, open, and ready for penetration without as much warm-up as usual.

A good plug will generally stay in place on its own. If not, a harness, G-string, or bondage tape can hold any toy with a flared base inside. And plugs with remote controls have limitless possibilities. If a top and bottom go out together while the bottom's wearing the plug, the top can take control of the remote and turn the vibrating toy on and off—making it extremely tough for the bottom to keep a straight face when talking to coworkers at a stuffy cocktail party!

FISTING

Let's dispel two myths about fisting right away. First of all, the term *fisting* is actually a bit of a misnomer. With fisting, the penetrative hand doesn't form a fist at all; it's more of a duckbill shape (although that doesn't sound very sexy!). Second, *fisting* sounds violent, but it's not. For most people, it's actually a very slow, intense, intimate, even spiritual activity that requires a lot of time, communication, and trust—especially for novices. That's because the anus has to open both physically and psychologically. While it'll still feel pleasurable, even seasoned fisters can't take a fist if their heads aren't into it. Plus, for both fister and fistee, the act can release plenty of endorphins and unexpected emotions, so both of you will want to proceed slowly and carefully. Here's how to start:

• Remove any rings from your fingers, and cut and file your fingernails; even if you're wearing gloves, the smallest nail or hangnail can damage the sensitive rectal lining.

• Clean yourself out ahead of time. Bits of fecal matter pressed and rubbed against the rectum with the intense pressure of an entire hand can be painful and can create tears in rectal tissue.

• Put down a towel or a disposable chuck—they're large, absorbent blue pads available in medical supply stores—to catch excess lube before it makes a mess of your sheets. (Using lots and lots of lube is vital. It feels great, and it allows a hand to slide in as easily as possible.) Crisco—yes, the kind used in baking!—and J-lube, which is used by veterinarians, are popular options for fisting, but they're not easy to clean up.

• Go slow. Fisting is not meant for quickies. Allow lots of time for arousal and to work up to a whole hand. Accomplished fisters may be able to open up in as little as 20 minutes, but most folks need 2 hours or more, especially for the first few times. Pressuring yourself to rush or to attain a goal will backfire. It's likely that your anus will close up rather than relax.

• Don't expect to take a whole fist the first time you try—or even the twentieth time. Some folks say that fisting is a lot like doing the splits or learning to ease into yoga poses. Each time you try, you'll probably relax and open more than you did the last time.

• Respect your body's boundaries. Don't push your body too far. Let it relax and open up at its own pace. Forcing yourself beyond your comfort levels can actually damage your sphincters or your rectal wall.

Very rough and prolonged anal sex is a big part of our kink, especially penetration with no lube or preparation, so initially it's very painful until the sphincters relax, and then it turns into extreme pleasure. We also do anal stretching and medical play with a speculum.

Before you try to take an entire fist, practice with toys of increasing diameters. Try thrusting and holding them in place for both short and long periods of time—but remember that thrusting can tire out your sphincters, while simply holding a toy in place can teach your body to relax against it.

After using a toy with a diameter of 3 inches (7.6 cm), you or your partner may be able to accommodate a fist. When the receiver is ready, insert one finger at a time. When you've inserted up to four or five fingers, rotate your hand in the direction of the butt crack, as though you were giving someone a handshake; your hand will slip in much more easily that way. Since your hand is in the shape of a duckbill, the knuckles on the back of your hand create a hump that may be difficult to insert. The knuckle on the back of the thumb presents a similar challenge. But once you slide the widest part of your hand past the sphincter, it'll move easily into the wider, more flexible part of the rectum while the anus relaxes against the narrower wrist. This sense of fullness is likely to feel intense in a different way. Your body is used to pushing things out when the rectum is full, and the same feeling will be triggered by a fist. When this happens, simply hold the fist in place without moving it. When your partner is ready for some additional sensation, limit your movements to small rotations of the wrist or hand, or gentle, slow, shallow thrusts.

With any type of intense anal play, muscle spasms are common. They're a natural way in which the body reacts to the sensations. Remain still and give the muscles time to relax. If your partner asks you to pull out, do so, but do it slowly. Removing a hand, toy, or penis too quickly can damage the sphincters.

After fisting, the lube in the anus might be tinged with pink. That's not uncommon: anal play can rupture capillaries, but this is rarely harmful. However, a bright-red color is a major warning sign. If this happens, stop what you're doing, and seek medical attention right away.

For more detailed information on anal fisting, see Bert Herrman's classic book *Trust: The Hand Book: A Guide to the Sensual and Spiritual Art of Handballing* (1991).

ELECTROSTIMULATION

Want to add a little electricity to your sex play—literally? Then electrostimulation might be right for you. Electrostimulators can be bought online for reasonable prices (try www.stockroom.com), and lots of folks like them because they arouse the muscles in the anal area, sphincters included. On low power, electrostimulation feels like a tickle; the higher the power, the more intense the tickle. (It can even feel like pins and needles, or cause muscle contractions!) Here's how it works. Lubricant conducts the electricity from the toy to your body. There are two points on each toy, and the electricity passes from one point to your body, then makes its way out through the other point. Beyond that, there are too many different styles of electrostimulation and safety precautions to list here, so if this type of play intrigues you, seek out good resources on safe electrostimulation, like Uncle Abdul's *Juice: Electricity for Pleasure and Pain* (1998), since it can be harmful and even dangerous if done improperly.

MIND PLAY

Mind games can be a good thing! If you get turned on by teasing and other psychological games, you might enjoy playing with the very same fears and myths surrounding anal play that we discussed in chapter 1. In his book *The Erotic Mind: Unlocking the Inner Sources of Passion and Fulfillment* (1996), Jack Morin, Ph.D., discusses the intense aphrodisiac effect that can arise from engaging with our fears. And Tristan Taormino outlines some of these techniques in her book *The Ultimate Guide to Anal Sex for Women* (2006). For example, if your partner is concerned about being dirty, telling her how filthy the toy, finger, or penis that just came out of her butt is might actually turn her on. Or if your partner says he's afraid of pain, you can elaborate on how much penetration will hurt (even when it won't) and tell him he won't be able to sit down for a week. When anal sex is taboo for your partner, you can build up the excitement by calling her or him a bad girl or bad boy for

enjoying anal pleasure. If this kind of "humiliation" play doesn't work for you or your partner, you can try other kinds of play. For instance, if your partner is struggling to accommodate a large toy, you can boost the anticipation by showing her a toy that's 2 inches (5 cm) wide—and then inserting the 1-inch (2.5-cm) toy instead while you tell her how good she's being.

Your brain is the most powerful sex organ you've got, so use it to make the most of kink and advanced anal play! Keep in mind, though, that each scene must be a turn-on for both partners. Anything short of enthusiastic consent can be psychologically and physically damaging. Take the time to reflect on your own kinks and to communicate your desires and boundaries with confidence. A lover who can articulate both his or her desires and her boundaries is easier to trust and to have fun with—so do your best to be that person!

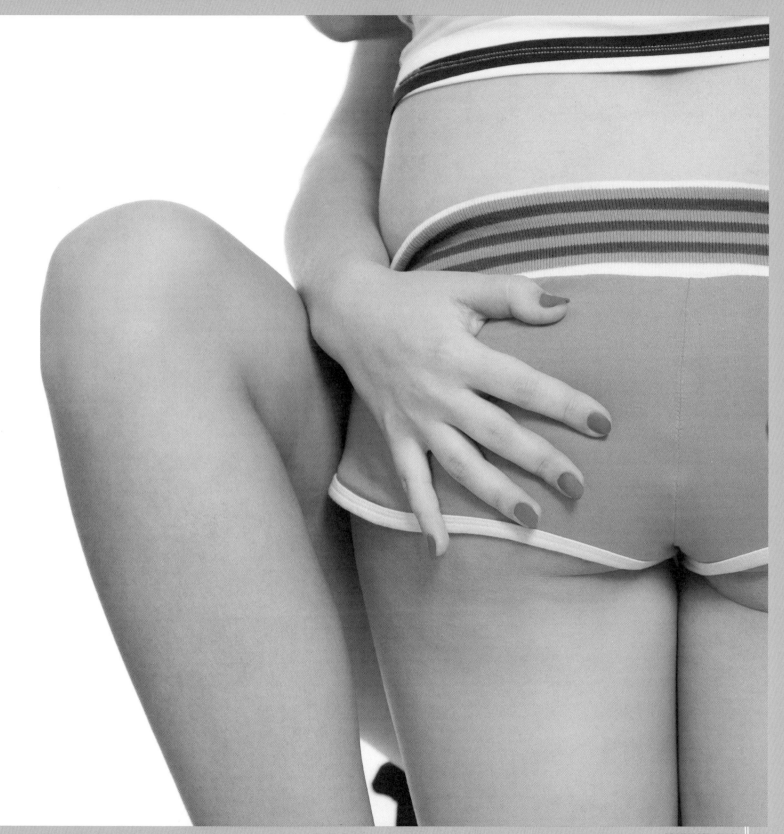

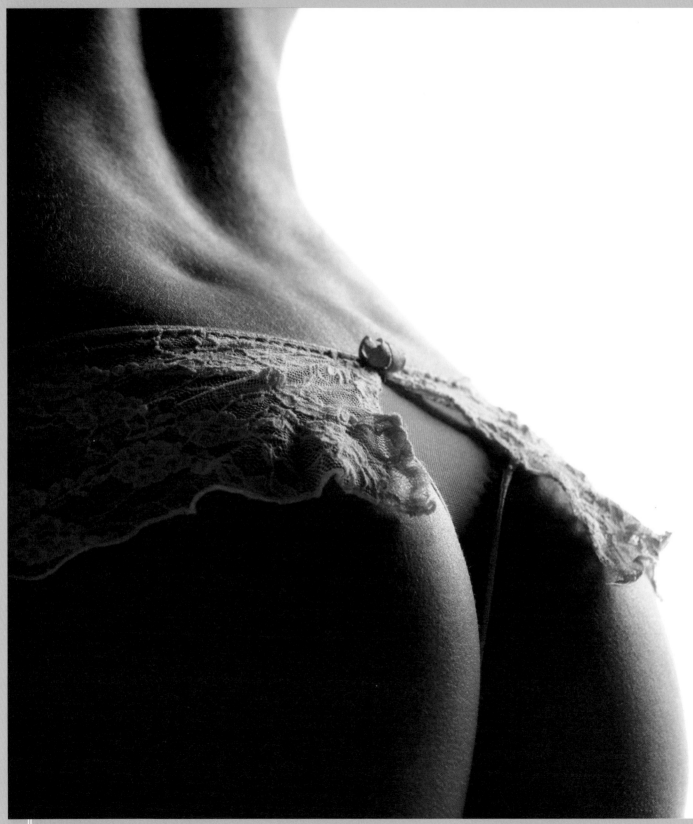

CONCLUSION

Thus ends our tour of the many anal options at your disposal. I hope you've learned a few new tricks to make your anal practice even better. You may be ready to delve into these more advanced possibilities, or perhaps you've decided that the basics are still the best choice for you. There is no right or wrong answer when it comes to choosing your path to anal pleasure. You get to decide what you want to do, how far you want to go, and when you want to stop. Wherever your adventures take you, don't forget the lessons you've learned:

1. Slow it down. Almost everyone who shared their experiences with me emphasized the need to slow down whatever you are doing in order to feel, listen, and enjoy the process.

2. Consider your goals. For most of us, a primary goal of sex is pleasure. If you manage to accomplish taking in a penis, toy, or one or more fingers, good for you! But hopefully that's not at the expense of pleasure, however you define it. Don't concern yourself with what others can do or enjoy. It's not a competition with your peers.

3. Lube! For pleasure and safety, use lots of it. And then add some more. Try a few brands until you find your favorite.

4. Start on the outside. If you plan on going inside, don't cheat the external nerve endings of your anus out of their own pleasure. Give them some attention, too, to warm you up— or just because it feels great.

5. Listen to your butt. It is smarter than you think. Don't try to force it to do anything it doesn't want to do. Pay attention to any pain, uncertainty, or limits that you reach to prevent tearing or harm to your body. Exert patience, and practice your technique to expand those limits, but don't forget that you'll need your butt's cooperation.

6. Communicate your desires. Don't be too shy to speak up about what you like and what you would prefer. There is no shame in asking for what you want. Just as importantly, be sure to listen carefully to your partner and heed his or her wishes.

7. Play safe. For each activity you choose to try, know its risks, no matter what type of relationship you enjoy with your partner. From prep to aftercare, plan your adventurous possibilities and start with the information and supplies you need to make it the best and safest possible.

8. Invest in proper toys. Always use toys with a flared base. Ask anyone who has worked in a hospital emergency ward about items retrieved from butts. The anal sphincters rarely work perfectly afterward.

9. Stick around. Especially if you played internally, give your body time to respond to the stimulation. Until you have experience with how your body reacts to butt play, it's prudent to stay close to a bathroom.

10. Be good to your butt. It's important to treat your butt well when you're not having sex, too. Eat well and adjust your diet if you are constipated. Don't put off your BMs if you can help it. Attend to hemorrhoids and other health concerns. You and your butt are partners for a lifetime!

REFERENCES AND RESOURCES

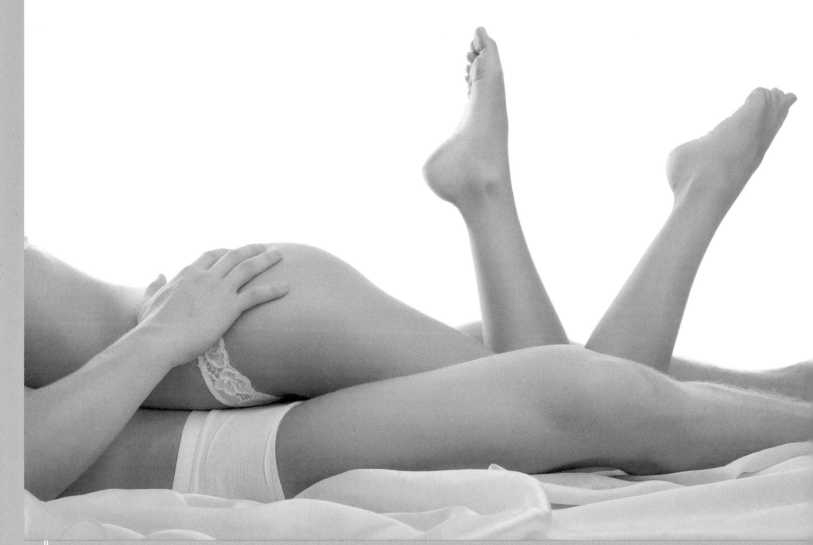

References

INTRODUCTION

Herbenick, D.; Reece, M.; Schick, V.; et al. (2010). "Sexual Behavior in the United States: Results from a National Probability Sample of Men and Women Ages 14–94." *Journal of Sexual Medicine* 7:255–65.

CHAPTER 1: MYTHS AND PLEASURES

Nickel, J.C. (1999). "Prostatitis: Evolving Management Strategies." *The Urologic Clinics of North America* 26(4):737–51.

CHAPTER 2: YOUR ANAL ANATOMY

Levitt, M.D.; Furne, J.; Aeolus, M.R.; Suarez, F.L. (1998). "Evaluation of an Extremely Flatulent Patient: Case Report and Proposed Diagnostic and Therapeutic Approach." *The American Journal of Gastroenterology* 93 (11):2276–81.

CHAPTER 3: GETTING READY FOR ANAL PLAY

Hussain, L.A., and Lehner, T. (1995). "Comparative Investigation of Langerhans' Cells and Potential Receptors for HIV in Oral, Genitourinary and Rectal Epithelia." *Immunology* 85(3):475–84.

Millett, G.A.; Flores, S.A.; Marks, G.; Reed, J.B.; Herbst, J.H. (2008)."Circumcision Status and Risk of HIV and Sexually Transmitted Infections among Men Who Have Sex with Men: A Meta-analysis." *JAMA* (Meta-analysis) 300 (14): 1674–84. doi:10.1001/jama.300.14.1674. PMID 18840841.

CHAPTER 8: TOYS, LUBES, AND CONDOMS

Rotello, G. (1996). "Our Little Secret." *The Advocate*, 705:72.

Beksinsta, M.E., et al. (January 2001). "Structural Integrity of the Female Condom after Multiple Uses, Washing, Drying and Re-lubrication." *Contraception* 63(l):33–6.

Resources

CHAPTER 3: GETTING READY FOR ANAL PLAY

Enemabag.com

CHAPTER 4: THE APPROACH

Joseph Kramer's *Anal Massage for Lovers* DVD

CHAPTER 5: TAKING THE PLUNGE

Mantak Chia's *The Multi-Orgasmic Man: The Sexual Secrets That Every Man Should Know* (2001).

CHAPTER 10: ADVANCED ANAL

Lord Morpheus (2015). *Bondage Basics.* Beverly, MA: Quiver Books.

Bert Herrman, *Trust: the Hand Book: A Guide to the Sensual and Spiritual Art of Handballing.*

GLOSSARY

BM
This is an abbreviation for bowel movement.

BOTTOM
This is a person receiving anal penetration and/or someone who enjoys being submissive to another in a BDSM/kink context.

CIS
Someone whose gender identity matches their biological sex is considered cis. For example, someone assigned female at birth who also identifies as a woman might identify as a cis woman

FLUID BONDED
When two partners share sexual fluids with each other but (if they have multiple relationships) use barriers for safer sex with others, they are considered fluid bonded.

INCONTINENCE
A person who is incontinent is unable to hold in his or her urine or BMs when desired.

PEGGING
This is an act whereby a woman penetrates a male partner's anus with a strap-on dildo.

PPG
In this book, this abbreviation is used to refer to prostate, perineal sponge, and/or G-spot stimulation in terms of the angle of anal penetration needed to effectively hit those areas.

RIMMING
This term refers to the stimulation of the anus with the mouth and tongue.

ROSEBUD
This is a non-anatomical name for the anus.

STI
A sexually transmitted infection is an infection passed onto another person often during sex; an updated term for STD or sexually transmitted disease, since many infections are curable and also to reduce stigma around having this type of infection.

TOP
This term refers to the person penetrating their partner anally and/or someone who enjoys taking control by dominating a partner who actively consents to it.

TRANS
A trans person is someone whose gender identity does not match their biological sex. For example, someone assigned female at birth might identify instead as a trans man or as simply trans (or many other terms as well) .

ACKNOWLEDGMENTS

A huge thanks to my first teacher, the late Chester Maynard, and to the Body Electric School, Collin Brown, Greg, and Michael, who helped me learn about butts in practical ways. I also want to acknowledge the pioneering work of the following authors: the late Jack Morin as well as Tristan Taormino, Bill Brent, Charlie Glickman, Aislinn Emirzian, and Sadie Allison. I am grateful to Joseph Kramer for expanding the potential of butt play to the masses, including myself. Many thanks also to all of my workshop participants and coaching clients at Good For Her, whose valuable feedback over the years has helped me understand what people actually want to learn.

Appreciation to Jon Pressick, Carey Gray, Phillip Coupal, Samantha Fraser, Andrea Zanin, ohd, and Tobi Hill-Meyer for adding their voices to the text.

Much gratitude to Dr. David Kennedy and Dr. Robert Chen for lending me their invaluable medical knowledge.

The many quotes throughout this book I owe to the awesome folks who took time to respond to my many questions: Toby B.D. Wiggins, Jon Pressick, Greg Wong, Stephen Biggs, Indira Dutt, Sade Petlele, Chrisanthi, Frances King, Julie Vix, Addi Stewart aka Malcolm Lovejoy, Tommy Hill, Mée Rose, Samantha Fraser, TL, Jenna, merpderp, Bievan, Phet, hungindallas, AMW, RD Australia, Gmanreno, Carley Mathews, reincatnated, SMG, ARS, JB (April), TLT, Erik Bergesen, and Bee.

Huge thanks to Megan Buckley and Jessica Haberman for their patience, spicing it up, and excellent editing. And huge hugs to my partner HK, my familiy, and everyone who has believed in me!

ABOUT THE AUTHOR

Carlyle Jansen is the founder of Good for Her, Toronto's premier sexuality shop and workshop center; author of *Sex Yourself;* and producer of the annual Feminist Porn Awards. Carlyle has been teaching workshops and coaching individuals and couples looking to enhance their sexual lives since 1995. She is passionate about education for everyone, and her teaching audience ranges from sexual health professionals and sex therapists to youth and parents, TV audiences, and informal groups of folks looking for fun ways to improve their sexual experiences. She is a regular contributor to *Tonic* magazine; has been featured in the *Toronto Star*, *Maclean's* magazine, *Globe and Mail*, and *Montreal Gazette;* and has appeared on the Discovery Channel, Women's Television Network, CBC, and many television stations and documentaries. She lives in Toronto, Canada.

INDEX

ALSO AVAILABLE

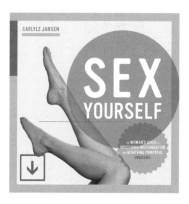

Sex Yourself
978-1-59233-679-1

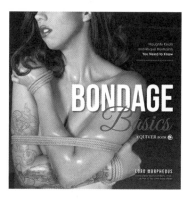

Bondage Basics
978-1-59233-645-6

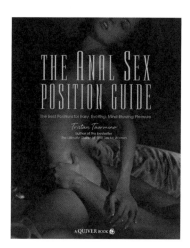

The Anal Sex Position Guide
978-1-59233-356-1

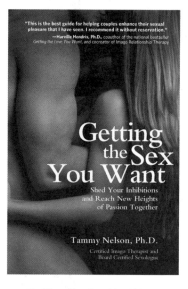

Getting the Sex You Want
978-1-59233-526-8